Advance Praise for *IBS-Free Recipes for*

"This book is filled with tasty recipes for dishes that kids ~~~~~ ~~~~ the *Whole Family* changed my 'tween daughter's attitude from dread to e ~~~~~ ~nn Miranda, *Executive Director & Co-founder, Fruitful Offerings*

"I found *IBS-Free Recipes for the Whole Family* to be more than a recipe book. It is also a good resource for a beginner or for someone already following a low-FODMAP diet. No matter how busy you are, or how unfamiliar with FODMAPs, this book will make your journey healthier and easier. Get ready to create delicious meals and snacks, learn how to navigate food labels and create a healthy pantry." – *Colleen Francioli, Certified Nutritionist Consultant, Founder, FODMAPLife.com and BonCalme.com*

"Finally...a family-friendly cookbook that everyone in the household can enjoy! Even better, this approach works!" – *Kasey Kaufman, Award-Winning Journalist and Filmmaker*

"This empowering book is a gift for IBS sufferers like me and for our loved ones who want to cook us meals we can enjoy together. I trust Patsy Catsos for accurate and easy-to-understand information about eating for IBS. I appreciate Lisa's compassion for families struggling to accommodate special diets; I am grateful for Karen's willingness to share her thirty-four years of experience working with children and families. This trio has blended their personal and professional expertise into an outstanding resource that belongs in your library next to Patsy's *IBS—Free at Last!*, which has become my gut health bible." – *Shalimar Poulin, recovering 15-year IBS sufferer*

"As a mom who has found relief with the low-FODMAP diet after years of discomfort and guesswork, cooking for my whole family had become a bit of a challenge. Thankfully, this cookbook has come to my rescue. It offers family-friendly and easy-to-prepare recipes that even my pickiest eater enjoys, and that is no small achievement. Now we're all happy!" – *Stephanie Carlson, OTR/L*

"This is a masterpiece that goes beyond the standard cookbook. Patsy Catsos, Lisa Rothstein, and Karen Warman provide a practical overview of the low-FODMAP diet with recipe substitutions that are quick and easy to follow. With creative and mouthwatering recipes, from appetizers, to main dishes, to side dishes, sauces, soups and even smoothies, there is definitely something for everybody. As a person who follows a low-FODMAP diet and a registered dietitian nutritionist, I am excited and inspired to try a new recipe from this book every day! I will also definitely be recommending this cookbook as a must-read and a keeper for my clients and their families." – *Ilene Cohen, MS, RDN, CDN, CDE, E-RYT, Owner, PranaSpirit Nutrition by Ilene Cohen*

IBS-Free Recipes for the Whole Family

Flavor without FODMAPs Cookbook Series

Lisa Rothstein, Patsy Catsos and Karen Warman

Foreword
by Athos Bousvaros, MD, MPH

This publication contains the opinions and ideas of its authors. It is sold with the understanding that the authors are not engaged in rendering medical, health, or any other kind of personal or professional services. Readers are urged to share the information in this book with a health care provider before adopting any of the suggestions. Readers are advised to discuss symptoms with a medical adviser and not to use this book to self-diagnose IBS. The authors and publisher specifically disclaim all responsibility for any liability, loss, or risk, personal or otherwise, incurred as a consequence, directly or indirectly, from the use or application of any of the contents of this book.

Copyright © 2015 Lisa Rothstein, Patsy Catsos, and Karen Warman

Pond Cove Press, P.O. Box 10106, Portland, ME 04104-0106

ISBN: 0-9820635-9-8

ISBN-13: 978-0-9820635-9-0

Cover image © Patsy Catsos

All rights reserved. No part of this publication may be reproduced, stored in a retrieval system or transmitted in any form or by any means, electronic, mechanical, photocopying, recording, or otherwise, without the prior written permission of the authors. Health care professionals have permission to photocopy up to four recipes for individual patient education.

Table of Contents

FOREWORD

Irritable bowel syndrome (IBS) affects 10 to 20 percent of Americans, and IBS isn't fun. At any point during the day, a patient with IBS may suffer from symptoms of bloating and abdominal pain, or get the urge to run to the bathroom. While IBS is not life-threatening, the symptoms can affect an individual's work life, sex life, and social life. If you don't believe me, just type the words "IBS sucks" into any internet search engine, and hear stories of patients afflicted with this condition.

As a gastroenterologist who specializes in the care of children and young adults, I often evaluate people with suspected IBS. Usually, patients come in with a history of gastrointestinal symptoms that have been occurring for several years. Many have had laboratory testing, which usually comes back normal. Some have been told the symptoms are "all in their head" (they're not). My usual approach to the patient with suspected IBS is to review prior studies, order additional blood work if needed, and screen for intestinal infections. Sometimes, more intensive testing (including x-rays, endoscopy, and colonoscopy) is needed to exclude conditions like celiac disease, Crohn's disease, and ulcerative colitis. If the history, examination, and lab studies suggest the likely diagnosis is IBS, I'll work with the patient to develop a treatment plan.

Treatment of IBS depends on the patient's symptoms, but usually involves a combination of medications, lifestyle alterations (e.g. stress reduction), and dietary modifications. One diet that has proven effective in treating some patients with irritable bowel syndrome is the low-FODMAP diet. FODMAP is an acronym given to a group of sugars and fibers (fermentable oligosaccharides, disaccharides, monosaccharides and polyols) that are commonly found in people's meals. While many individuals can handle these without difficulty, some people with IBS have trouble tolerating them, leading to the debilitating symptoms of the condition. Controlled studies suggest that some (but not all) patients who go on a low-FODMAP diet exhibit symptom improvement compared to patients who stay on their regular diet.

How does this diet work? No one knows exactly, but in most IBS patients it's probably NOT a food allergy. More likely, low-FODMAP diets work by altering the intestinal microbiome (the trillions of bacteria that live inside your intestine). Recent medical research suggests that IBS patients may develop their symptoms because they have different bacteria living in their intestine compared with patients without IBS. Such bacteria might ferment foods differently, produce more gas, and alter the intestine's motility, resulting in either diarrhea or constipation. By reducing the amount of FODMAPs ingested, and reducing the "fuel" for these potentially harmful bacteria, an IBS sufferer can control his or her symptoms.

There's one catch: a low-FODMAP diet isn't easy. These sugars and fibers are common in our Westernized diets, including foods such as milk, beans, apples, and various condiments. High-fructose corn syrup is a high-FODMAP sugar that is frequently used in processed foods. Because these foods and ingredients are so commonly found in supermarkets and restaurants, an IBS patient who wants to practice a low-FODMAP diet needs to be adept at reading labels and preparing foods. The following book, prepared by two experienced registered dietitian nutritionists and a creative recipe developer, is a wonderful guide towards living a low-FODMAP lifestyle. The helpful information and recipes will serve as a useful guide to any person who wants to treat IBS with this approach.

In summary, a low-FODMAP diet is not a guaranteed "cure" for IBS, and it is not right for everyone, but it helps many patients. As with any medical intervention, please make sure your health care team knows you are trying this approach, and consider using it in conjunction with other tools such as medication and stress relief. We hope reading this book will lead to a healthier, happier you!

Athos Bousvaros, M.D., M.P.H.
Associate Professor of Pediatrics, Harvard Medical School
Associate Chief of Gastroenterology, Boston Children's Hospital

INTRODUCTION

Lisa's Story

Diagnosed with IBS in my teens, I spent years trying a myriad of recommended diets, probiotics, and exercise, but nothing seemed to help. As years passed the symptoms waxed and waned, but as I got older and followed the mantra of health experts to "RELAX! EAT MORE FIBER! EAT MORE FRUITS AND VEGETABLES! EAT MORE YOGURT!" my symptoms became constant and more severe. One day at a weight-lifting class, I met dietitian Karen Warman, and we became workout partners. Between sets we discussed food, cooking, nutrition and health, all passions of mine. Karen mentioned that as a nutritionist she counseled patients with IBS at her clinic, and I opened up to her about my struggles. I knew that certain foods were causing my IBS because when I ate very little my symptoms would drastically subside. However, I could not find a pattern or connection between specific foods and the symptoms. Karen mentioned that she had had a lot of success with patients on the low-FODMAP diet plan. She explained the diet, gave me several research papers, and mentioned the book, IBS—Free at Last! by Patsy Catsos, as a resource. I was skeptical but desperate to feel better, so I plunged into learning more about it. I was shocked that the low-FODMAP foods recommended were completely opposite to the ones my health care providers and other IBS self-help books claimed would help my condition. No wonder I always felt worse following their advice! While the research papers on the low-FODMAP diet made sense to me scientifically (I am a former research scientist), much of the online information was sketchy and conflicting. The book IBS—Free at Last! was easy to follow, and it was the key to finding the right direction. As someone who loves food, I initially panicked when I read about the food restrictions. Nevertheless, I started eating low-FODMAP foods and eliminating high-FODMAP ones, and within a week my IBS symptoms were drastically reduced. Two weeks later, I felt like I was getting my life back.

Never one to fear a cooking challenge, and not willing to feel deprived, I rolled up my sleeves, made new grocery lists, and began a frenzy of cooking, baking, and writing down new recipes. Before long I had over 150 recipes that I knew were not just healthy, but tasted great to me and my family. I wondered how others who were not as comfortable cooking as I was would fare with this daunting new way of eating. Online comments made me sad when people trying low-FODMAP diets lamented that they were eating plain boiled chicken and white rice. In my mind I yelled, "You don't have to!!!" I decided I needed to share my recipes with others who might be struggling with this diet so they could feel as good, and eat as well, as I did. And so this cookbook idea was born. Karen and I decided to work on the project together. Because Karen works in pediatrics and I was cooking not just for myself, but also for my children and husband, we decided to focus on family-friendly recipes.

Serendipitously, Karen and Patsy were seated at the same table a few months later at a professional event in Chicago, where they were both attending the International Celiac Disease Symposium hosted by the University of Chicago. That meeting led to Karen and me contacting Patsy for a potential collaboration. Uncannily, when Patsy and I met for the first time, we each showed up with a plate of home-made low-FODMAP cranberry-orange scones to offer the other! Our collaboration seemed fated, and it blossomed from that point forward into this cookbook. I wrote and developed all of the recipes in the cookbook. Karen and Patsy, as nutrition professionals with years of clinical experience between them, wrote the non-recipe portions of this book. I'll turn the remainder of this introduction over to them!

FODMAPs Come into Their Own

Since the first edition of *IBS—Free at Last!* was published in 2009, the low-FODMAP approach has risen to the top of the list of effective dietary treatments for irritable bowel syndrome (IBS). While still not a household word, FODMAPs have been covered by the *New York Times, Web MD, Huffington Post, Glamour, Fox News, Redbook, The New Yorker, Dr. Oz, Living Without, More*, National Public Radio and other major outlets. Adult and pediatric doctors are recommending the diet more than ever. FODMAPs, which are certain sugars and fibers in food that can cause gastrointestinal distress for people with IBS, were the cover story of the January, 2014, edition of *Gastroenterology*. Scientific evidence for the effectiveness of the low-FODMAP diet continues to accumulate, and many more studies are underway. Is "FODMAPs" the new hot diet? Is it a healthy, long-term diet for everyone? No! Low-FODMAP diets should be reserved for use as a short-term, dietary experiment for people with irritable bowel syndrome, to help determine which foods are well-tolerated and which are not. Nutritious high-FODMAP foods should only be eliminated long-term if absolutely necessary to manage symptoms.

How This Book Can Help You and Your Family

If your doctor or nutritionist asks you or a family member to try a low-FODMAP diet, you will quickly encounter a few problems:

- There are a limited number of commercial products available that match the requirements of the diet.
- You need recipes for family-friendly foods that everyone will enjoy.
- You may have concerns about whether you are getting all the nutrients you need from your diet.
- Not everyone in the family needs to be or should be on a low-FODMAP diet.

This book was written to help address these concerns. We provide ideas for quick and easy foods as well as some that are more adventurous for the budding foodie, all of which can be enjoyed by the whole family. The recipes avoid high-FODMAP ingredients that are known to worsen symptoms such as excess gas, bloating, diarrhea, constipation, and abdominal pain. Only one recipe in the book (Seitan Breakfast Sausage) deliberately contains gluten, so gluten-free eaters will be able to easily use this recipe collection. People with lactose intolerance or dietary fructose intolerance (also known as fructose malabsorption or FM) will also be able to use these recipes, all of which are low in lactose and fructose.

It is not the intention of this book to re-write *IBS—Free at Last!* by Patsy Catsos, which provides a detailed, step-by-step plan for undertaking a FODMAP-elimination diet. It is not the intention of this book to replace individualized advice and guidance from your own health care providers. Rather, this is a family-oriented cookbook, with some helpful information about making the FODMAP approach work in a family setting. Whether you are using this book for a child who has been advised to follow a low-FODMAP diet or you are an adult (with IBS) with children in your life, the meals you prepare will be shared by family and friends. To successfully incorporate a low-FODMAP diet into family life, you need to meet the needs of those with dietary restrictions while still pleasing the palates of reluctant family members. This book offers a much needed jump-start to that process.

It's critical that you understand there isn't a lot of science to go on for use of low-FODMAP diets with children (just one small pilot study and one small, short-term randomized clinical trial). In fact, one of the important goals of this book is to offer appropriate cautions about over-enthusiastic use of this or any other restricted diet in a household with children. However, we know that as a parent you can't wait 10 years for all the science to be in when your child has a tummy ache today. Parents are trying to help by restricting the diets of their children, with or without our input, and pediatric specialists are recommending the low-FODMAP diet for children. We'd like to share helpful information for those families without promoting inappropriate use of the diet.

We can't say it too often: make sure your family member with symptoms of abdominal pain, excess gas, bloating, diarrhea, and/or constipation gets a proper evaluation by a qualified health care provider. Meet with a registered dietitian nutritionist with expertise in the use of low-FODMAP diets; get a referral from your physician or see the list of dietitians participating with your insurance company. Use this cookbook to prepare meals the whole family can enjoy. Finally, draw upon all of your sensitivity and tact to help the person with IBS feel better physically while fostering harmonious family relationships and confident food choices.

Food Trends and FODMAPs

Why are so many Americans (up to 20% of us) experiencing symptoms of IBS significant enough to prevent us from enjoying or fully participating in our usual activities, such as school, work, and play? Scientists are still trying to understand the underlying cause of IBS. However, there is quite a bit of scientific evidence suggesting that the community of bacteria in the guts of IBS sufferers is out of balance. At the same time, carbohydrates that feed bacteria are finding their way into our food supply in increasing amounts. Certain high-FODMAP ingredients on the "avoid" list are new within the past 40 years, thus significantly increasing the FODMAP content of our food supply. Some of them have been added for economic reasons, such as high-fructose corn syrup, which makes food cheaper to produce. Others have been added for perceived health reasons, such as inulin to increase fiber content or sorbitol to reduce added sugars.

High-fructose corn syrup (HFCS) was introduced into the US food system in the 1970s when cane sugar became less available from certain countries due to political reasons. It quickly caught on with food manufacturers, and high-fructose corn syrup is now used for a variety of purposes in foods, including as a flavoring agent, to improve texture, for browning baked products, as a preservative, and to enhance fermentation. The actual fructose content of different types of high-fructose corn syrups varies. HFCS found in baked goods is slightly lower in fructose than that used in beverages. Although we saw a significant increase in HFCS from 1970 to 2000, there is a now a trend toward removing it from products. We now find some manufacturers clearly labeling their products "no high-fructose corn syrup." Fructose itself is now frequently added in pure form to foods. It is used frequently in chewable supplements, protein powders, and beverages, which can be labeled "all-natural" or "no artificial sweeteners."

Inulin is a fiber found naturally in food including chicory root, artichokes, onions, and garlic. Inulin is a "prebiotic." That means it feeds bacteria. Prebiotics provide nourishment to more than 5,600 different species of bacteria found in the human gastrointestinal tract. Research shows that nourishing good bacteria in the gastrointestinal tract improves digestion and enhances mineral absorption for most people. This finding, in addition to the fact that most Americans do not consume enough fiber, has encouraged food manufacturers to add inulin or chicory root to many foods. In fact, inulin is pretty well tolerated by people with healthy guts, causing just a minor increase in flatulence. Unfortunately, for people with IBS, consuming inulin or chicory root can result in a bout of IBS symptoms. Research shows that inulin extracted from chicory root results in more symptoms than when inulin is naturally present in foods. Carefully read the labels of foods that advertise "improved digestion," "more fiber," or "lower calories." Inulin, chicory root, and other new-fangled fibers will show up in the list of ingredients if they are present. They can be found in certain (not all) herbal teas, protein shakes or powders, yogurt, cottage cheese, cream cheese, sweeteners, kefir, puddings, frozen desserts, quick-cooking rice, multi-grain or gluten-free bread, breakfast cereal, instant oatmeal. We have even seen it in bottled water! Since there is a source of organic chicory root, reaching for a product labeled organic will not exclude the addition of inulin. If you see more grams of fiber listed on the nutrition facts panel than there would normally be in a similar product, double check those ingredients!

Sorbitol, xylitol, and mannitol are "sugar alcohols," also known as polyols (the "P" in FODMAP). These sugar alcohols are added to foods as low-calorie sweeteners and to help keep foods moist. Because they are slowly and incompletely absorbed, they provide fewer calories than sugar and have less effect on blood sugar. While this might be desirable for diabetics, it can aggravate symptoms for people with IBS. Sugar alcohols are added to certain (not all) brands of sugar-free candy, ice cream, chewing gum, mints, cough drops, pancake syrup, cakes, cookies, and low-carbohydrate bars. They are also found in certain liquid or chewable medications, vitamins, minerals, and other supplements. The Food and Drug Administration requires labeling of products that contain more than 50 grams of sorbitol or 20 grams of mannitol with a warning that "excess consumption may have a laxative effect," but some individuals are sensitive to much smaller amounts, and laxation isn't the only problem these ingredients can cause. Note that these products are actually natural because they are derived from plants. So avoiding so-called "artificial" sweeteners won't do the trick.

Larger portion sizes across the board are another food trend driving our increased intake of FODMAPs in the United States. This is true both in the home, where enormous dinner plates have become the norm, at restaurants and at the supermarket. Bigger portions contribute more FODMAPs and can leader to more dramatic bouts of IBS symptoms.

Some of us have changed the way we eat in what we hope is a healthier direction. But certain dietary improvements can be "too much of a good thing" for people with IBS. Examples of seemingly healthy (but high-FODMAP) choices include unlimited fruits and vegetables, lots of milk or yogurt, smoothies, protein powders, juicing, trail mix, nutrition bars, high-fiber multi-grain breads, and raw, plant-based or vegan diets. It may be frustrating that the more you try to improve the family's diet, the more trouble you (or your child) may have with excess gas, bloating, and abdominal pain. These are actually clues that the FODMAP approach might help.

UNDERSTANDING THE FODMAP APPROACH

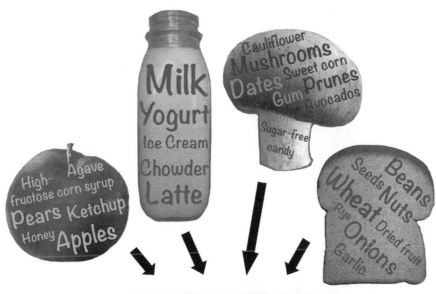

FODMAPs are certain sugars and fibers in your diet.
All FODMAPs from your diet go into the
same "bucket."

What Are FODMAPs?

Is the term "FODMAP" new to you? If so, you are not alone. FODMAP is the acronym for **F**ermentable **O**ligo-, **D**i-, and **M**onosaccharides **A**nd **P**olyols. Don't let this awkward term scare you away. You don't have to be a biochemist to eat a low-FODMAP diet. We've studied the science so you don't have to. Here are the important parts:

FODMAP carbohydrates include certain natural *sugars* in foods such as milk, fruit, honey, and high-fructose corn syrup. FODMAPs also include certain *fibers* in foods such as wheat, onions, garlic, and beans. (Speaking of wheat, note that gluten is not a FODMAP—it's just a coincidence that FODMAPs and gluten coexist in wheat, as well as in rye and barley.) The load of FODMAPs from all sources has a cumulative effect. That means your overall FODMAP intake from a variety of sources matters. Examples of FODMAPs are:

- Lactose (also known as milk sugar, found in milk, yogurt, and ice cream)
- Fructose (also known as fruit sugar, found in fruit, high-fructose corn syrup, honey, and agave syrup)
- Sugar alcohols such as sorbitol, mannitol, and other "-ol" sweeteners (found in certain fruits and vegetables, as well as some types of sugar-free gum and candy); sugar alcohols are sometimes known as polyols
- Oligosaccharides (sometimes referred to as fructans and GOS) are short-chain fibers found in wheat, onions, garlic, chicory root, beans, hummus, and soy milk

How Do FODMAPs Trigger Symptoms?

All FODMAP carbohydrates have a few things in common:
- They may be poorly absorbed in the small intestine. Instead, as the hours go by after a meal, these sugars and fibers linger in the small intestine, then move along into the large intestine.
- They are the favorite foods of the normal bacteria that live in the intestines. When these bacteria eat FODMAPs, a process called fermentation creates a lot of gas.
- FODMAPs can act like a sponge to pull extra water into the gut and disrupt fluid balance.

With a little imagination, you can picture the combination of gas and fluid causing the intestines to swell up like a water balloon. People with IBS experience this as a painful bloating sensation. They may pass an excessive amount of gas (flatulence, wind, or farts) or have urgent watery diarrhea, constipation, or both.

People who do not have IBS may not be bothered at all by eating FODMAPs. Bacterial fermentation is actually a normal part of life and produces some substances that are valuable to our health. The intention of the FODMAP elimination and challenge process is not to stamp out fermentation altogether, but to keep it at a manageable level.

Who Should Try a Low-FODMAP Diet?

The best candidates for low-FODMAP diets can answer "yes" to the following questions:
- Do you have digestive symptoms such as excess gas, bloating, abdominal pain, diarrhea, and/or constipation?
- Have you been properly evaluated by a health care professional and diagnosed with IBS or another condition that might benefit from a low-FODMAP diet?
- Has your doctor or dietitian recommended a FODMAP-elimination diet?
- Has celiac disease been ruled out?
- Have you been unable to manage your symptoms with good health habits like regular meals, managing stress, and getting adequate amounts of fiber, fluids, and exercise?
- Are you physically, mentally, and emotionally able to limit your diet for a period of time without endangering your health?

- Are you willing and able to take on a dietary experiment?

Some people may not be good candidates for an elimination diet, including people with inflexible eating habits, those who are medically, mentally or emotionally fragile, those who are at risk for eating disorders, and those who do not have full control over their food purchasing and preparation. These individuals are strongly advised to work with a registered dietitian nutritionist, who may be able to recommend medically appropriate changes informed by the FODMAP approach without requiring a full-fledged elimination diet. *In addition, diet changes should be delivered with great sensitivity and tact to children.*

Risks and Benefits of Low-FODMAP Diets

The effectiveness of the low-FODMAP diet has been demonstrated by careful studies conducted by a team at Monash University in Australia. Researchers Susan Shepherd and Peter Gibson published their first scientific paper about FODMAPs in 2005. Since then, controlled trials in the hands of other researchers from New Zealand and England have shown similar results. The benefits are clear for adults: up to 75% of adult IBS sufferers get significant and long-lasting relief of symptoms from a low-FODMAP diet.

A small pilot study of low-FODMAP diet in eight children demonstrated a trend toward reduced abdominal pain, although the differences were not statistically significant. A somewhat larger follow-up study by the same group at Baylor College of Medicine compared IBS symptoms in a group of children who ate two days of low-FODMAP diet followed by two days of a typical American childhood diet or vice versa. The children reported significantly fewer episodes of abdominal pain on the low-FODMAP diet than on the typical American childhood diet. Pain severity also decreased significantly on the low-FODMAP diet compared to the children's baseline scores. Other IBS symptoms were not significantly different. These results vary from numerous adult studies, which have showed significant improvements in all IBS symptoms on low-FODMAP diet. Why the difference? Two days may not have been long enough for the children to get the full benefit of the diet. A particularly well designed adult study found that maximum symptom relief was achieved after an average of seven days on a low-FODMAP diet. The study results also may have been affected by a high dropout rate among study participants.

Clinical studies typically focus on whether or not the treatment effect on the group *as a whole* was statistically significant. One drawback of this traditional approach is that it intentionally overlooks individual differences in the response to the treatment. In this case, the Baylor researchers were able to identify significant difference in the distribution of gut bacteria present in the stool of the eight children who responded to the low-FODMAP diet versus the 15 children who were non-responders. Responders had more bacteria capable of fermenting carbohydrates. This intriguing finding, if replicated, could eventually improve our ability to predict the best candidates for the FODMAP approach. Clearly more research will be necessary before we can draw broad conclusions about the benefit of the diet for the pediatric IBS population as a whole, but these early studies are encouraging and it is apparent that some individual children do have a strong response to the diet.

It is important to note that a FODMAP elimination diet has some potential risks. Prebiotic intake is reduced on a low-FODMAP diet. (Prebiotics are food for the good bacteria that are part of a healthy gut microbiome.) Research has shown that adopting a low-FODMAP diet reduces the bacterial load in the colon. This includes a reduction in what are presumed to be beneficial bacteria. So far, no negative health consequences related to this have been demonstrated. Still, people who do not have a medical reason to try a low-FODMAP diet should not do so.

Eating a low-FODMAP diet can affect nutrient intake unless care is taken to choose a wide variety of low-FODMAP foods. Not all of the changes are bad, but some concerns have been raised. In one study, adults following the diet had lower intake of total carbohydrates, starch, total sugars, and calcium. There is a wide range of acceptable carbohydrate and starch intake, and a lower intake of sugar isn't a bad thing, but reduced calcium intake is a potential problem. Another study compared the nutrient intakes of three groups of people. One group had IBS and had received guidance on the low-FODMAP diet two years earlier. The second group had IBS but patients were *not* on a special diet. The third was a group of healthy people. There was no significant difference between the three groups in overall intake of calories, total carbohydrates, proteins, fat, or sugar. The bad news was that "unguided" patients with IBS had low intake of several important nutrients compared with healthy people, partly because they chose to consume fewer milk products. The good news was that IBS patients who were guided on the low-FODMAP diet did better than the other IBS patients at keeping up their intake of essential nutrients like potassium, magnesium, calcium, B vitamins, and beta-carotene. The guidance we would like to pass along to you is this: there are plenty of good sources of all necessary nutrients in your low-FODMAP pantry. If you choose and eat a wide variety of low-FODMAP grains and starches, fruit, vegetables, proteins, and fats, your nutrient intake is very likely to be just fine.

Very picky eaters or those who recognize that they are unwilling to try nutrient-rich alternatives to high-FODMAP foods should seek assistance from a dietitian before trying the diet. If you choose to avoid certain food groups (vegetarians and vegans) or can't tolerate a wide variety of low-FODMAP foods, you've got to work harder at monitoring your intake of nutrients, especially protein, fiber, and calcium. See our chapter Meeting Your Nutrition Needs, beginning on page 27, for help with those nutrients. Many of the low-FODMAP breads and cereals made from alternative grains are not fortified or enriched with thiamine, niacin, riboflavin, iron, or zinc, placing these nutrients in a "watch" category to assure adequate intake.

If one person in a family is following a low-FODMAP diet, should family members with healthy guts eat low-FODMAP recipes? Sure! Eating food made from low-FODMAP recipes is not bad for other people as long as their total diet still has a wide variety of healthy higher-FODMAP fruits, vegetables, nuts, seeds, and whole grains. Lactose-free cow's milk products are just as nutritious as regular milk and yogurt. There's nothing nutritionally unique about wheat, so eating less of it won't hurt the rest of the family. Anyone's health can benefit from less added sugar. More homemade food is likely to elevate the family's diet, if anything, and other family members can easily add high-FODMAP extras to their own plates or to other meals of the day as needed. Pass the chopped onions in a separate bowl to sprinkle on the salad, and everyone will be happy.

What to Expect on a Low-FODMAP Diet

A FODMAP elimination diet is a temporary learning diet; it is not meant to be a permanent way of eating. It is important to have realistic expectations: the diet will not cure IBS, because FODMAPs aren't the underlying cause of IBS. FODMAPs are not bad in and of themselves. The problem, which is still poorly understood, is the way the gut of someone with IBS *responds* to consuming FODMAPs. You can expect to learn whether changing your intake of FODMAPs will help you manage your IBS symptoms. At first you will choose and eat only low-FODMAP foods, such as the ones in the Low-FODMAP Pantry section of this book. You will learn more from this experience if you stick closely to the foods in your Low-FODMAP Pantry during the first few weeks. Consider upcoming trips, holidays, and special events already on the calendar—start the diet during a few weeks when you can spend some extra time on planning, shopping, and food preparation.

You should start to feel better within a few weeks if your symptoms are related to FODMAPs. How will you know if the diet has worked? It's your call. There are no blood or stool tests that will tell you if it worked, which FODMAPs are causing your symptoms, or how much FODMAP-rich food you can eat without getting symptoms. The learning process depends entirely on your observations about what happens when you remove and then reintroduce FODMAPs (sometimes called the challenge or re-challenge phase of the diet).

If you achieve symptom relief on the low-FODMAP diet, you may want to just enjoy it for a few weeks. Many of our patients say they've never felt better! But soon, ideally with the guidance of your dietitian, FODMAP-containing foods can and should be re-introduced. By paying close attention to your symptoms, you will learn which FODMAPs are triggers for your IBS (so you can limit or avoid them), as well as which ones you are able to tolerate. You will learn the most from the approach if you follow a disciplined process for reintroducing FODMAP-containing foods to your diet. Detailed guidance on the elimination and re-challenge process is outside the scope of this book. Seek help from a knowledgeable registered dietitian nutritionist or see www.ibsfree.net for links to other publications that can assist you.

Your eventual goal is to eat the most varied and nutritious diet that you can tolerate. We encourage you to do the best you can to reintroduce *valuable* high-FODMAP foods when you are ready. Do we care if you ever have high-fructose corn syrup again? No, not really. It adds nothing to your nutrient intake but empty calories, and may use up some of your capacity to tolerate other, more valuable foods. High-FODMAP whole fruits, vegetables, and beans, on the other hand, have a lot to offer, and we hope that if you find you can tolerate only limited amounts of FODMAPs, you choose these foods over sweets, fruit juice, and baked goods. One common criticism of books like this is the lack of detailed guidance on the process of reintroducing FODMAPs. We hear you, but it can't be helped! The process of reintroducing FODMAPs will be as individual as you are. Some people (those with small intestinal bacterial overgrowth, severe IBS symptoms or anxiety) will need to proceed with caution and others will take a gung-ho approach to challenging themselves with larger intakes of their favorite foods. Some people will be intolerant of just one or two types of FODMAPs and some people will have to keep their load of FODMAPs from all sources low or moderately low. Keep these points in mind:

- Eat a wide variety of low-FODMAP foods.
- Work at liberalizing your diet as much as you can. Don't stay on a low-FODMAP diet for longer than you must. If you find you don't have a problem with some types of FODMAPs, don't continue to restrict them after the first few weeks. Modify these recipes in reverse. Add back at least a few of those onions. Garnish with a few raisins. Drink regular milk and eat Greek yogurt again if you can. Commercially made broth and salad dressing might be fine for you if you can handle some onions and garlic.
- Prioritize nutrition-rich, higher-FODMAP foods. Limited ability to tolerate FODMAPs is like being on a budget. Spend your FODMAPs wisely on high-priority foods. Splurge on one or two higher-FODMAP foods a day if that's all you can manage.
- Keep your FODMAP load under control by choosing naturally lower-FODMAP foods or by choosing only small portions of high-FODMAP foods. Love pizza? Develop a taste for thin crust pizza, have just one slice, and hold the onions. Love beans? Have a spoonful or two in your minestrone soup instead of a whole bowl full of bean soup. Love Greek yogurt? Go ahead and try some. It contains just a few grams of lactose, and you may do just fine with one serving a day.

One nice thing you can expect from a low-FODMAP diet is a new appreciation for homemade food and cooking from scratch. Many of our adult patients tell us they wish they had been taught more cooking skills as children or young adults; they have been forced to rely on heat-and-serve foods and takeout for many years! Involve the children in the planning and preparation of meals and don't be afraid to admit that you are all learning together. Cooking from scratch is often cheaper, gives you full control over the ingredients that go in your food, and passes along valuable knowledge and skills to the next generation. This is a good time to roll up your sleeves, gather helpful family members around you and make baking and cooking together a new family activity.

Using the FODMAP Approach with Children

In this section we will discuss some specific concerns related to using the FODMAP approach with children, including how being on a special diet can affect relationships with parents, siblings, and friends. The most important message is to proceed with caution and only with the input of your child's doctor and dietitian, who will help you judge whether the benefits of trying the diet outweigh the potential risks. Be sure to discuss how the child will communicate whether or not the diet is working.

Being on a special diet has some social and psychological impact. A sense of feeling left out or not being able to fully participate in food-related events is sometimes reported by patients in our practices. For the school-age child, you can handle this by planning ahead and making suitable food choices available (see Planning Meals for the Whole Family on page 35). For the early adolescent (ages 12 to 14), this presents a bigger problem, as they often don't want help from a parent and at the same time want to fit in without appearing to be different. Teens and preteens who have been advised to try the diet will probably find it less stressful if they understand the rationale for the diet. Be sure to communicate that it truly is an experiment and not a permanent life sentence. They won't have to give up pizza forever. What they learn from trying the diet will be worth it: it will ultimately give them more control over their lives and make them more independent.

Make sure your child does not misunderstand the use of the word diet, which is often used to refer to weight-loss programs. This diet is not about losing weight, just about choosing different foods for a few weeks to see if it helps manage IBS symptoms.

For all ages, it helps a great deal socially if you can make low-FODMAP food that friends and family are able to enjoy along with the "patient," which is no doubt why you are reading this cookbook. We know that it's a little difficult to change the way you are used to operating in the kitchen. You can acknowledge this with your child and the rest of the family as well. Many of your family's usual foods may contain high-FODMAP ingredients like regular flour and milk, onions, garlic, ketchup and soft drinks. However, if those foods are resulting in discomfort to someone in the family, it is time to find new meals and recipes that can be enjoyed together as part of new family traditions. It's important: research has found parents in families that eat together on a regular basis are more likely to know what is going on in their children's lives. This leads to improved behavior and health as nutrient needs are more likely to be met.

Some children are at greater psychological risk than others from a restricted diet of any type. Anxious younger children might benefit more from having the food supply at home quietly change in the low-FODMAP direction without so much as a single discussion. It may be difficult for younger children to switch gears from "we're not eating apples this week" to "apples are OK again." Please do *not* label or refer to FODMAP-containing foods as "bad foods" or "bad for you." It just isn't true for most foods, and it will be confusing and anxiety-provoking when you ask your child to try eating these foods again. Don't overreact if your child makes a mistake or even purposely makes an exception during a trial of the low-FODMAP diet. It's true you will both learn more the closer your child sticks to the low-FODMAP foods at first, but the whole project isn't ruined by a mistake or exception, and he or she might even learn something from it. We usually advise young people to do the best they can to choose low-FODMAP foods in every eating situation, but not to go hungry if nothing suitable is served.

Let's face it, adolescence is a high-risk age for disordered eating, and gastrointestinal complaints can be part of anorexia nervosa or bulimia. If there is *any question* in your mind whether your teen or preteen might be at risk for an eating disorder, do not encourage him or her to try any type of restrictive diet. Instead, discuss your concerns with your child's physician, who can refer you to appropriate providers for guidance. Eating disorders can be life-threatening; IBS is not. Protecting your child from unintentional weight loss (which can trigger an eating disorder all by itself) and from developing a fearful relationship with food is more important in the long run than perfect adherence to a low-FODMAP diet.

What about picky eaters? Entire volumes have been written about picky eaters and how to manage them. We recommend speaking with your pediatrician about this problem, which is beyond the scope of this book. Dietitian and family therapist Ellyn Satter is the foremost American expert on parenting healthy eaters. Her books, *How to Get Your Kid to Eat: But Not Too Much* and *Child of Mine: Feeding with Love and Good Sense,* offer wise counsel on preventing and managing feeding problems in young children. The Ellyn Satter Institute is widely hailed as a helpful resource by pediatric specialists. *Just Two More Bites! Helping Picky Eaters Say "Yes" to Food* by dietitian Linda Piette is worth reading. Finally, parents of children whose picky eating threatens their health should consult the book, *Food Chaining: The Proven 6-Step Plan to Stop Picky Eating, Solve Feeding Problems and Expand Your Child's Diet*, by medical professionals Cheryl Fraker, Mark Fishbein, Sibyl Cox and Laura Walbert. Children whose picky eating rises to the level of a serious behavioral problem, who would rather starve to death than eat some fresh berries instead of drinking a box of apple juice, are probably not good candidates for the FODMAP approach.

It's interesting to note that the concept of special children's menus or "kid-friendly foods" emerged only in the last 50 years. The term is often used to describe bland, easy-to-eat food like chicken nuggets, macaroni and cheese, pasta, and pizza. In fact, this cookbook project got its start because we needed low-FODMAP versions of such foods to suit the preferences of our young patients. While these foods are not necessarily bad as part of an overall healthy diet, relying on them every night will result in a lack of variety in the diet. Children and adolescents need nutrients from a variety of foods to continue to grow and develop. For that reason, in this book we challenge you to cook with a wider range of fresh, whole foods. These recipes have been well-received by many children, including our own, even though they are not on the typical children's menu.

Prior to beginning the low-FODMAP process, it is important to scrutinize your child's symptoms. Think about both the type of symptoms and the degree of impact that they are having on his or her life. Discuss the plan for monitoring symptoms with your child's health care team. Parents of young children should take responsibility for observing and documenting symptoms, preferably with a minimum of discussion. We know that increased attention to symptoms may reinforce them. Sometimes children will agree that they are having symptoms (whether they do or not) if asked leading questions. On the other hand, it will be frustrating if you go to the effort of trying the diet, relying on your child's ability to state whether he or she feels better or not, and the response is "I don't know." Adolescents often take more ownership of the process when they track their own symptoms and see results from making changes in their diet.

You might try using a scale to track symptoms such as abdominal pain (cramps, bellyache), excess gas (farting, wind), bloating, distension (visibly bigger belly), nausea, urgency to use the toilet, feelings of incomplete evacuation (like you need to have a bowel movement even though you just had one), diarrhea (frequent, mushy, or watery stools), constipation (difficulty pooping, hard, dry stools, or infrequent bowel movements), and fatigue. Do not run through this litany of symptoms every time; only inquire about symptoms your child has reported to you. Ask simple yes or no questions or make up a smiley face scale like the one on page 12. Low-key inquiries about symptoms once a day should be adequate to determine a baseline and whether the diet is working without getting over-involved in every little sensation your child feels in the gut. We need to avoid creating the impression that feeling our digestive system working is necessarily a bad thing! Passing gas is certainly normal and sometimes even people without IBS are extra gassy at times, or feel a strong intestinal signal prior to a bowel movement. It is also normal for stool form and frequency to vary somewhat from day to day. As tempting as it is to keep track of "objective" data like the number of bowel movements per week or per day or how often we pass gas, these numbers are often not as relevant as any associated pain, discomfort, or impact on our ability to attend work or school.

		Overall, how did you feel?	Symptom:	Symptom:	Symptom:
🙂	No symptoms today 1				
🙂	Aware of gut 2				
😐	Mild symptoms; easy to ignore 3				
😕	Few bouts of moderate symptoms 4				
😟	Moderate symptoms all day 5				
☹️	Symptoms severe at times 6				
😫	Terrible day; missed usual activities				

The same questions or scale should be used again after a time on the low-FODMAP diet to help you decide if the diet is working. Did the diet improve your child's sense of well-being? Did improved bowel habits and less abdominal pain allow fuller participation in school, work, sports, and social life? Were the necessary diet changes worth the improvement in symptoms? It's a judgment call. There is no blood test or X-ray that will make this decision for you or your child. If the low-FODMAP diet is a big improvement, you probably owe it to your child to stick with it for a while as you learn more about what happens when you try testing his or her tolerance to reintroduced FODMAPs. Think about the symptoms you are monitoring again as you do so, and rate them using the same questions or scale. Keep in mind that high-FODMAP foods may not result in symptoms for hours or even until the next morning, and that the more the child eats, the greater the odds of developing symptoms and the greater the possible severity of those symptoms. This will help you determine whether symptoms were related to the intake of FODMAPs and the degree of restriction necessary for your child to have a good quality of life. What if your child doesn't want to stick with aspects of the low-FODMAP diet, even though it helps? Will FODMAPs damage his or her health? We have no evidence to suggest that continuing to consume FODMAPs from otherwise-healthy foods causes any actual physical damage to your child's body, so you don't have to worry about that. Perhaps you can negotiate limiting FODMAP intake for a few days prior to important events or family activities, so they will go more smoothly. If your child knows symptoms can be managed as needed with FODMAPs, he or she always has a safe place to go with diet.

YOUR LOW-FODMAP PANTRY

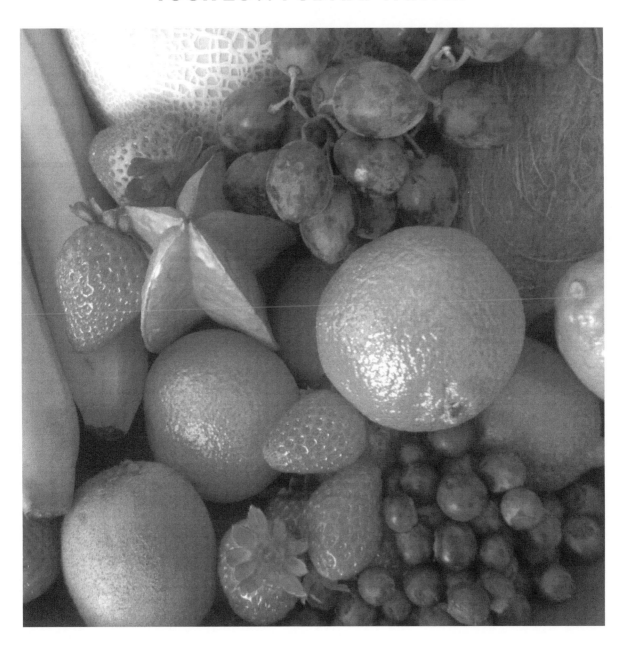

How to Use Your Low-FODMAP Pantry

To pull off a successful FODMAP elimination diet, you've got to have low-FODMAP foods on hand when it's time to make your next meal. Stock your pantry and refrigerator with some of these staples, and you'll be prepared. In all cases, buy a brand that does not contain FODMAP ingredients. For example, *jam* is in the pantry, but it must be jam made from low-FODMAP fruit such as blueberries and sweetened with a low-FODMAP sweetener like sugar. Mustard is in your pantry; at the time of this writing, French's Classic yellow mustard contains garlic powder, so a better choice would be Annie's Naturals Organic Yellow Mustard. Because manufacturers change ingredients frequently, please read the label *every time* to check for FODMAPs. Ingredients and brand names change frequently, so we have not listed brand names in the pantry. Here are some things that might help:

- We've placed an asterisk (*) after the items that often contain FODMAP ingredients and are your highest label-reading priorities. These are all processed foods. The easiest way to make sure your foods don't contain FODMAPs is to choose the fresh whole foods listed instead of food that comes in bottles, cans, or boxes.

- Patsy has developed a Pinterest board with low-FODMAP, brand-name grocery items at www.pinterest.com/pcatsos. When you view Patsy's Pinterest boards, you can see pictures of brand-name groceries that are likely to be suitable for a low-FODMAP diet based on her review of the ingredients. Few of them have been laboratory tested for FODMAPs.

- A variety of apps and web sites can help you read the ingredients of grocery items online, which might make planning an easier task. Some of our favorites are Shopwell.com, Foodfacts.com, and Fooducate.com. Many grocery store chains also have websites with ingredient lists for an extensive array of products. Focus on the list of ingredients on these sites and apps; the rating systems were designed with other considerations in mind and do not relate directly to the low-FODMAP diet.

Some of the foods in the pantry will be new to you. You don't have to eat them if you don't want to, especially if you are doing a short-term elimination diet. However, if you find yourself following a low-FODMAP diet over a more extended time period, these alternative foods can expand your culinary horizons. A more varied diet offers a wider variety of nutrients, too.

Some of the items in your low-FODMAP pantry do have small amounts of FODMAPs in them. For best results, you should only eat one or two portions of those foods at a time; **look for the bold font and note the recommended portion.** Other (non-bold) foods can be consumed according to your caloric needs and appetite. The recommended portion sizes are geared toward older children, teens and adults. They are based on clinical experience, not research, but we think you will agree that they are small portions, perhaps half the portion size that many people might normally choose. If you are using this diet with a younger child, think about what that child's normal portion of the "bold" food would be and cut it in half. For example, if you would normally serve your child 10 grapes, you should serve him or her 5 grapes while doing a low-FODMAP diet. Don't forget to increase portions of the non-bold foods to keep calorie intake up to appropriate levels.

Be sure to modify these food lists to suit your other health conditions. For example, people with gluten-related disorders should not eat foods containing gluten, such as sourdough bread, and should use only gluten-free versions of foods on this list such as oats, breakfast cereals, tempeh, and soy sauce. There are many other conditions, too numerous to list, that require dietary modification. Please seek help from a registered dietitian nutritionist to modify these food lists as needed.

Gluten, Sourdough Bread, and Your Low-FODMAP Pantry

The Grains and Starches section of your low-FODMAP pantry needs some special introduction. If you are new to FODMAPs you might need help fully understanding the distinction between gluten and FODMAPs in wheat and wheat products. If you are familiar with FODMAPs, you might be surprised to see the inclusion of several new wheat-based foods on this list of foods which are suitable for the elimination phase of the diet.

First of all, we'd like to remind you that the FODMAP approach is a short-term dietary experiment to learn about how *FODMAPs* in food may be affecting your IBS symptoms. We understand that IBS is complicated and that FODMAPs are not the only dietary components that might affect your gastrointestinal health. In fact, we encourage you to work with a dietitian to modify this diet according to your individual concerns; the whole point of the FODMAP approach is finding the diet that is right for you; there is no one-size-fits-all diet for IBS. Dietitians are trained to respect and help all patients with their nutrition needs, not just those who share our own food preferences or lifestyle. As dietitian-authors, if our book is based any food philosophy at all, it is this: you should eat the most varied and nutritious diet you can tolerate, consistent with your own food preferences.

This leads us to the subject of gluten and FODMAPs. We are aware that some enthusiasts of the FODMAP approach say low-FODMAP diets must be gluten-free. That is not true for most people. By definition, all FODMAPs are carbohydrates. Gluten is not a carbohydrate; it is a protein. Therefore, gluten is not a FODMAP and a low-FODMAP diet does not have to be gluten-free. Is it possible to do a gluten-free version of the diet? Yes, it is relatively easy to do, because many gluten-free grains and starches are naturally low in FODMAPs as long as high-FODMAP ingredients have not been added during processing or preparation. In fact, only one recipe in this book deliberately contains gluten (Seitan Breakfast Sausage). Might it be a good idea to do a gluten-free version of the diet? The answer to that question will be different for each person. Here are a few scenarios to discuss with your health care team when deciding whether to modify the food lists in your Low-FODMAP Pantry.

- If you have a gluten-related disorder such as celiac disease or dermatitis herpetiformis, you should choose only gluten-free foods. Gluten-containing foods are not marked in this book, to keep the focus on FODMAPs. *However, please note that sourdough breads are not gluten-free and are not safe for those with celiac disease.*

- If you believe yourself to have non-celiac gluten sensitivity you might consider avoiding gluten at first, but we encourage you to reintroduce it at some point to test tolerance. Because wheat, barley and rye are sources of both gluten and oligosaccharides, many people whose gastrointestinal symptom improve on a gluten-free diet may be benefiting from consuming fewer FODMAPs; the gluten may have nothing to do with it.

- If you are allergic to wheat, do not eat wheat in any form.

- If you don't have a diagnosed gluten-related disorder or non-celiac gluten sensitivity, use the Grains and Starches food list as written.

In August, 2015, Monash University released an update to the Low FODMAP Diet app indicating that sourdough breads made of white flour, whole wheat flour and spelt flour are low in FODMAPs. We think this is great news! Traditionally made sourdough breads taste great and are the closest low-FODMAP alternative to regular bread. Ordinary breads made of these flours are not typically low in FODMAPs; they contain oligosaccharides. What makes sourdough breads different?

The difference lies in the techniques used for rising, or "proofing," the bread. Commercially made breads contain baker's yeast and some kind of sugar. Baker's yeast quickly ferments the sugar, and the bread dough is proofed and ready for baking in just a few hours. On the other hand, traditional sourdough bread-making uses a complex mixture of yeasts and lactic-acid forming bacteria carried over from the last batch of bread (a "starter") to ferment, develop and proof the dough over an extended time, from many hours to days. Bacteria in the starter break down the oligosaccharides to sugars, and the yeasts consume the sugars, eventually producing enough carbon dioxide gas to make the bread rise. In short, the microbes in the starter consume oligosaccharides in the bread dough, reducing its FODMAP content.

It can be difficult to identify authentic sourdough breads in the marketplace. The bread-making process, not the sourdough flavor, is the key. Calling a bread "sourdough" does not necessarily make it so. You might find real sourdough bread in the bakery section of a well-stocked supermarket, but probably not in the bread aisle with all the ordinary, soft-crusted breads. It should have a chewy crust and a mild tangy flavor. Authentic sourdough breads do not typically include baker's yeast in the list of ingredients (the yeast itself isn't the problem but is a clue to rapid proofing). Sourdough breads do not contain preservatives, so they have shorter shelf lives and tend to come from local bakeries. You may even be able to discuss the bread-making process with the local baker who supplies the supermarket. If you are eating a lot of sourdough bread on your low-FODMAP diet and not getting significant symptom improvement, cut back on it or try another brand.. If that doesn't help, eliminate sourdough bread and try a gluten-free version of the diet.

Grains and Starches

Breakfast cereals, cold, made of amaranth, rice or corn, ½ cup*
Breakfast cereals, cold, made of quinoa or millet*
Buckwheat groats and flour
Corn or tortilla chips*
Corn pasta
Corn starch
Corn tortillas, 6-inch*
Cornmeal
Crackers, rice or corn*
Gluten-free bread, white, 2 slices (60g)*
Gluten-free pretzels*
Grits
Millet and millet flour
Millet bread*
Oat bran, dry, 1 tablespoon
Oat flour, ¼ cup
Oatmeal, ¼ cup dry or ½ cup cooked*
Plaintain

Polenta
Popcorn*
Potato chips*
Potato starch
Potatoes, white
Quinoa pasta
Quinoa, quinoa flakes,* and quinoa flour
Rice bran
Rice cereal, hot
Rice crackers*
Rice or popcorn cakes*
Rice pasta
Rice, brown, white, basmati
Sorghum and sorghum flour
Sourdough bread, white, wheat or spelt, 2 slices (90g)*
Tapioca starch
Teff flour
Wild rice
Yam flour

Tip: Avoid seasoned grain mixes; they usually contain onion or garlic.
* Read the label and avoid processed foods that have FODMAP ingredients added.
Bold: Contains a small amount of FODMAPs. For best results, do not exceed the portion size shown.

Fruits

Banana, ½
Blueberries, ½ cup
Blueberry juice, ½ cup
Cantaloupe, ½ cup
Clementine, 1 medium
Coconut water, ½ cup
Coconut, shredded, ½ cup
Cranberries, raw, ½ cup
Cranberry juice, ½ cup*
Dragon fruit, ½ cup
Durian, ½
Grape juice, ½ cup
Grapes, all kinds, ½ cup

Honeydew, ½ cup
Kiwi, 1 medium
Mandarin, 1 medium or 2 small
Orange juice, ½ cup
Orange, 1 small
Papaya, ½ cup
Passion fruit pulp, ½ cup
Pineapple, ½ cup
Prickly pear fruit, 1
Raspberries, ½ cup
Rhubarb, ½ cup
Star fruit, 1 medium
Strawberries, ½ cup
Tangelo, 1 medium

Tips: Limit fruit to one serving per meal or snack, 3-5 hours apart. Choose fresh or frozen fruit. No dried fruit or fruit juice drinks; no fruit juice other than those listed.
* Read the label and avoid processed foods that have FODMAP ingredients added.
Bold: Contains a small amount of FODMAPs. For best results, do not exceed the portion size shown.

Vegetables

Alfalfa sprouts
Arugula/rocket
Bamboo shoots
Bean sprouts
Bell peppers, green, yellow, orange or red
Bok choy, ½ cup
Butternut squash, ½ cup
Cabbage, common or red, ½ cup
Carrots
Celeriac/celery root, ½ cup
Chayote
Cherry tomatoes
Chicory leaves
Chile pepper, red
Choy sum
Collard greens
Cucumber
Eggplant
Endive
Fennel bulb, ½ cup
Green beans, ½ cup
Kabocha squash

Kale
Leaf lettuce
Leek, leaves only
Okra, ½ cup
Parsnip
Pattypan squash
Pickle, dill or sour
Pumpkin, canned, ½ cup*
Radicchio
Radishes
Scallions/green onions, green part only
Seaweed/nori
Spaghetti squash
Spinach
Summer squash
Sweet potato, ½ cup
Swiss chard
Tomato, fresh
Tomatoes, canned, whole, diced, crushed or pureed*
Turnip/rutabaga, ½ cup
Water chestnuts
Zucchini

Tip: Choose fresh vegetables or frozen vegetables without sauce.
* Read the label and avoid processed foods that have FODMAP ingredients added. Verify canned tomato products do not have added onion or garlic.
Bold: Contains a small amount of FODMAPs. For best results, do not exceed the portion size shown.

Nuts and Seeds

Almond butter, 2 tablespoons*
Almonds, 2 tablespoons
Brazil nuts, 2 tablespoons
Chestnuts, 2 tablespoons
Chia seeds, 2 tablespoons
Hazelnuts, 2 tablespoons
Macadamia nuts, 2 tablespoons
Peanuts, 2 tablespoons

Peanut butter, 2 tablespoons*
Pecans, 2 tablespoons
Pine nuts, 2 tablespoons
Poppy seeds, 2 tablespoons
Pumpkin seeds/pepitas, 2 tablespoons
Sesame seeds, 2 tablespoons
Sunflower seeds, 2 tablespoons
Walnuts, 2 tablespoons

Tip: Choose raw or roasted, unseasoned nuts and seeds. Two tablespoons equal one small adult handful.
* Read the label and avoid processed foods that have FODMAP ingredients added.
Bold: Contains a small amount of FODMAPs. For best results, do not exceed the portion size shown.

Oils

Coconut cream, canned, ½ cup
Coconut milk, canned, ¾ cup
Margarine
Mayonnaise*
Oil, all types, including olive, soybean, canola, peanut, safflower, corn, vegetable, coconut, sesame and garlic-infused
Tartar sauce*

* Read the label and avoid processed foods that have FODMAP ingredients added.
Bold: Contains a small amount of FODMAPs. For best results, do not exceed the portion size shown.

Milk Fats

Butter
Half-and-half, 2 tablespoons
Heavy cream, whipped, ¼ cup*
Sour cream, 2 tablespoons*
Sour cream, lactose-free

* Read the label and avoid processed foods that have FODMAP ingredients added.
Bold: Contains a small amount of FODMAPs. For best results, do not exceed the portion size shown.

Meat/Fish/Poultry/Eggs

Beef	Fish, any kind
Buffalo	Goat
Chicken	Lamb
Duck	Pork
Egg whites	Seafood, any kind
Egg, whole	Turkey

Tip: Choose unseasoned, unbreaded, and minimally-processed or ground meat, fish, and poultry.
* Read the label and avoid processed foods that have FODMAP ingredients added.

Plant-Based Proteins

Chana dal, cooked, ½ cup*
Chick peas, canned, drained, rinsed ½ cup
Lentils, canned, drained, rinsed, ½ cup
Tempeh*
Tofu*

Tip: Choose medium, firm, or extra-firm tofu that has been pressed and drained; silken tofu is not suitable.
* Read the label and avoid processed foods that have FODMAP ingredients added.
Bold: Contains a small amount of FODMAPs. For best results, do not exceed the portion size shown.

Cow's Milk and Milk Products

Cheese, American, 1 ounce
Cheese, hard, regular or reduced-fat including
    Cheddar, Swiss, Parmesan, Brie, mozzarella,
    feta, Romano, Havarti, Camembert
Cottage cheese, lactose-free*
Cream cheese, 2 tablespoons*

Dry curd cottage cheese
Goat cheese/chèvre , 1 ounce
Kefir, lactose-free*
Milk, lactose-free
Yogurt, lactose-free*

* Read the label and avoid processed foods that have FODMAP ingredients added.
Bold: Contains a small amount of FODMAPs. For best results, do not exceed the portion size shown.

Beverages

Almond milk, 8 fluid ounces*
Beer
Black tea, weak, 8 fluid ounces
Chai tea, weak, 8 fluid ounces*
Coffee, black, filtered or instant
Dandelion tea, weak, 8 fluid ounces*
Espresso, black

Green tea
Hemp milk, 8 fluid ounces*
Peppermint tea
Spirits (not rum)
White tea, 8 fluid ounces
Wine, red or white (not sherry or port)

Tip: Alcohol and caffeine can affect gut function even in low-FODMAP beverages; consume in moderation.
* Read the label and avoid processed foods that have FODMAP ingredients added.
Bold: Contains a small amount of FODMAPs. For best results, do not exceed the portion size shown.

Sweets

Brown rice syrup, 1 tablespoon
Candy/chocolate made with allowed
    ingredients, 1 ounce*
Cane syrup, 1 tablespoon
Chocolate, dark or semi-sweet, 1 ounce*
Corn syrup (not high-fructose), 1 tablespoon
Golden syrup, 1 tablespoon

Ice cream, lactose-free, ½ cup*
Jam or jelly, 1 tablespoon*
Maple syrup, 100% pure (not "pancake" syrup), 1
    tablespoon
Sorbet, ½ cup*
Sugar: light brown, cane, palm, confectioner's,
    granulated, demerara, raw, 1 tablespoon

* Read the label and avoid processed foods that have FODMAP ingredients added.
Bold: Contains a small amount of FODMAPs. For best results, do not exceed the portion size shown.

Condiments and Seasonings

Allspice
Asafetida
Basil
Bay leaf
Black pepper
Capers
Cardamom
Chile pepper, whole or ground
Chives and garlic chives, green part only
Cilantro
Cinnamon
Cocoa powder, 1 ½ tablespoons
Coriander
Cumin
Curry leaves
Curry powder*
Dill
Fennel seeds
Fish sauce
Five spice
Garlic-infused oil (without garlic "extract")
Ginger
Ground chiles (100% chiles, not a blend)
Italian seasoning*
Lemon
Lemongrass

Lime juice
Marjoram
Miso paste
Mustard seeds or powder
Mustard, prepared*
Nutmeg
Olives
Oregano
Oyster sauce, 1 tablespoon
Paprika
Parsley
Poultry seasoning*
Rosemary
Saffron
Salt
Scallions, green part only
Sesame oil, toasted or spicy
Soy sauce
Stevia
Tamari*
Tarragon
Thyme
Turmeric
Vinegar, balsamic, 1 tablespoon
Vinegar, other types
Wasabi*

Tip: Choose single-ingredient fresh or dried herbs.
* Read the label and avoid processed foods that have FODMAP ingredients added
Bold: Contains a small amount of FODMAPs. For best results, do not exceed the portion size shown.

Sugar and low-FODMAP diets

Sugars that are considered suitable for low-FODMAP diets contain *less* fructose than honey, agave, and high-fructose corn syrup. However, they are not fructose-free. If you over-eat sweets, you may be consuming more fructose than you can handle, and symptoms can result. You may also be cheating yourself out of the nutrition you could be getting from more valuable FODMAP-containing foods.

Think of your overall capacity to tolerate FODMAPs as your "budget" for the day. If you spend your budget on too much chocolate or brown sugar or too many servings of the dessert recipes in this book, you might find you can never get beyond the lowest FODMAP vegetables, nuts, fruits, grains or beans. That is a real loss in terms of both nutrition and your food quality of life.

If you are using the low-FODMAP diet because you have been diagnosed with small intestinal bacterial overgrowth (SIBO), please discuss with your doctor or dietitian whether you should be using any added sugar at all during your treatment.

LABEL READING

The most important part of the food label for people on low-FODMAP diets is the list of ingredients. If you are on the elimination phase of a low-FODMAP diet, choose only products with low-FODMAP ingredients. *That is not to say they are all "healthy choices," and we are not endorsing their use by listing them here.* What's right for one person may not be right for another. For example, while we don't endorse the use of aspartame, we are sharing the information about its FODMAP status with you so you can make an informed decision about whether or not you want to consume it. Likewise, gluten or sucralose may have effects on GI function, but they are not FODMAPs. That's right, gluten is not a FODMAP, and a low-FODMAP diet does not have to be gluten-free, despite what you may read elsewhere, although many gluten-free foods happen to be suitable for the diet. Of course, you may choose to omit any of these ingredients or additives if you wish. With the exception of salt, which provides the nutrient sodium, none are essential parts of the diet. If in doubt, please discuss appropriate choices with your dietitian.

Low-FODMAP Ingredients

Aspartame
Baker's yeast
Baking powder
Baking soda
Bar sugar
Barley malt
Beet sugar
Berry sugar
Black pepper
Brown rice syrup
Brown sugar
Cane juice crystals
Cane sugar
Cane syrup
Carageenan
Caster sugar
Cocoa butter
Confectioner's sugar
Corn syrup (not high-fructose)
Corn syrup solids
Cornstarch

Cultured corn syrup
Dehydrated sugar cane juice
Demerara sugar
Dextrose
Gelatin
Gellan gum
Glucose
Gluten
Granulated sugar
Guar gum
Gum acacia
Gum Arabic
High-maltose corn syrup
Icing sugar
Invert sugar
Malt extract
Maltodextrin
Maltose
Modified food starch
Organic sugar
Palm sugar

Partially hydrolyzed guar gum (PHGG)
Pectin
Raw sugar
Refined sugar
Resistant starch
Saccharine
Salt
Soy lecithin
Soybean oil
Stevia
Sucralose
Sucrose
Sugar
Sugar syrup
Superfine sugar
Tara gum
Vital wheat gluten
Wheat starch
Whey protein isolate
Xanthan gum

Label reading on the low-FODMAP diet is tricky. The degree to which ingredients must be avoided changes, depending on where you are in the process, and what your level of tolerance is to the ingredient in question. **The focus of this book is on succeeding with the elimination phase of the diet.** This phase is the strictest, and complete avoidance of high-FODMAP ingredients is recommended. If the FODMAP ingredient appears anywhere in the list of ingredients, avoid that product. None of the recipes in this book use high-FODMAP ingredients.

However, please keep in mind that a FODMAP elimination diet is meant to be a short-term learning diet, not a permanent way of eating. While some of these foods are no great loss nutritionally speaking, many of them contain valuable nutrients. After a few weeks on a low-FODMAP diet, make an effort to reintroduce higher-FODMAP vegetables, beans, whole grains and fresh or frozen fruit as tolerated. The best way to do this is to follow a reintroduction schedule designed to help you figure out your level of tolerance to each type of FODMAP. Details on that process are outside the scope of this book. Please visit Patsy's website, www.ibsfree.net, for resources, including a directory of registered dietitian nutritionists familiar with the FODMAP elimination and challenge process and links to her book, *IBS—Free at Last!*

Traces of high-FODMAP ingredients such as wheat or soy do not disqualify a product from being suitable for a low-FODMAP diet. For example, soy sauce often has wheat ingredients, but it is low in FODMAPs. A millet bread might have been made on equipment that also processes wheat bread, but if no wheat flour is actually on the list of ingredients it is suitable for a low-FODMAP diet. Unlike the diet of someone with a classic food allergy or celiac disease, the low-FODMAP diet does not have to be 100% free of all traces of the ingredient to be avoided. Simply avoid foods that deliberately contain them as ingredients.

A few disclaimers: Please note that the following is not a complete list of foods that contain FODMAPs, because our knowledge base is still incomplete. There can be discrepancies between the specific foods listed on various teaching tools. These can occur when tools become outdated or because the creators of the tools make different choices about portions sizes or cut-offs for what is considered high-FODMAP. Cut-off levels for FODMAPs are based on clinical experience and have not yet been validated in clinical trials. We do NOT recommend the following foods and ingredients during the elimination phase of a low-FODMAP diet.

High-FODMAP Foods and Ingredients

Agave nectar
Agave syrup
All-purpose flour
Amaranth flour
Apple cider
Apple juice
Apple sauce
Apples, fresh or dried
Apricot nectar
Apricots, fresh or dried
Artichoke hearts
Artichokes
Asparagus
Avocado
Baked beans
Barbecue sauce made with high-fructose corn syrup
Barley and barley flour
Beets
Biscuits made with wheat, barley, or rye flour
Black beans

Blackberries
Boysenberries
Bread made with barley or rye flour
Bread made with spelt flour (unless sourdough)
Bread made with wheat (white or whole wheat, unless sourdough)
Breakfast bars
Broccoli
Brussels sprouts
Bulgar wheat
Butter beans
Buttermilk or buttermilk solids
Cakes made with wheat, barley, or rye flour
Candy, made with high-fructose corn syrup
Candy, sugar-free, made with "-ol sweeteners"
Cannellini beans
Cappuccino, unless made with lactose-free milk

Carbonated soft drinks made with high-fructose corn syrup
Carob powder
Cauliflower
Celery
Celery salt
Chamomile tea
Cherries, fresh or dried
Chicory root or extract
Chocolate, white or milk
Coconut milk beverage
Cookies made with wheat, barley, or rye flour
Cottage cheese, unless lactose-free
Cough drops, sugar free, made with "-ol" sweetener
Couscous, unless made of rice
Crackers made with wheat, barley, or rye flour or grains
Crystalline fructose

Dates
Dried fruit
Dry milk solids
Eggnog, unless lactose-free
Enriched flour
Erythritol
Evaporated milk
Fennel leaves
Fennel tea
Fructooligosaccharides (FOS)
Fructose
Fructose solids
Fruit juice concentrates
Fruit punch or fruit juice cocktail made with high-fructose corn syrup
Garlic
Garlic powder or flakes
Garlic salt
Glycerin
Goat's milk, unless lactose-free
Green peas
High-fructose corn syrup
Hydrogenated starch hydrolysates
Inulin
Isomalt
Jam or jelly sweetened with high-fructose corn syrup, juice concentrates, or high-FODMAP fruits
Kamut
Kefir, unless 99% lactose-free
Ketchup made with high-fructose corn syrup
Kidney beans
Lactitol
Lattes, unless made with lactose-free milk
Leeks, white part
Lima beans

Low-carb or "net-carb" bars
Macaroni, white or whole wheat
Maltitol
Mango, fresh or dried
Mannanoligosaccharides(MOS)
Mannitol
Milkshakes
Milk, unless lactose-free
Molasses
Muffins made with wheat, barley, or rye flour
Mushrooms, fresh or dried
Natural flavorings (in cases which may refer to onions or garlic)
Navy beans
Nectarines
Non-fat dry milk
Oat milk
Oatmeal bread
Onions
Onion powder or flakes
Onion salt
Oolong tea
Orzo, white or whole wheat
Pancake syrup made with high fructose corn syrup
Pasta, white or whole wheat
Pesto made with garlic
Peaches, fresh or dried
Pear juice
Pears, fresh or dried
Pinto beans
Pistachios
Plums, fresh or dried
Polydextrose
Preserves made with high-fructose corn syrup or high-FODMAP fruits
Pretzels made with wheat, barley, or rye

Prune juice
Prunes
Rice milk
Scallions, white part
Seasoned salt
Semolina flour
Shallots
Snow peas
Sorbitol
Soy crumbles
Soy milk made from whole soy beans
Spaghetti, white or whole wheat
Spelt flakes
Spelt flour (unless in sourdough bread)
Spelt pasta
Split peas (except chana dal)
Sprouted wheat
Sprouted wheat bread
Sprouted wheat bread
Sugar snap peas
Sweet corn, fresh, frozen, canned
Tahini
Texturized vegetable protein
Tomato paste
Veggie burgers
Watermelon
Wheat berries
Wheat bran
Wheat flakes
Whey protein concentrate, unless 99% lactose-free
White flour (unless in sourdough bread)
Whole wheat flour (unless in sourdough bread)
Xylitol
Yogurt, unless lactose-free

Label Reading Practice

After the first few weeks of the low-FODMAP trial, previously "avoided" ingredients and foods can be reintroduced to determine tolerance. At that point, it is useful to note that ingredients are listed on food labels in order by weight. The ingredient contributing the most weight to the product is listed first, then in descending order down to the ingredient that weighs the least, which will be listed last. Reading the list of ingredients will not tell us how many grams of FODMAPs are in the food, but can give us a rough idea of whether or not the ingredient is present in a large or small amount. Other claims or information about the food, such as "fresh," "organic," "gluten-free," or "natural" are irrelevant as far as FODMAPs are concerned. For example, gluten-free foods often work on this diet because they don't have wheat, barley, or rye in them, but they could contain other high-FODMAP ingredients such as inulin or pear juice concentrate, so you must still read the label. Organic foods can't contain high-fructose corn syrup because there is no organic source of that ingredient, but organic foods can still contain many other kinds of FODMAPs. Almost all FODMAPs are considered natural.

Try out your label-reading skills on the following exercises by comparing the ingredients to those in the preceding lists. We know that some of the ingredients are not addressed on either the low- or high-FODMAP ingredient lists, but you should still manage to figure which product in each grouping is probably lower in FODMAPs, even with incomplete information—that's real FODMAP life.

Which of the following cottage cheeses is probably lower in FODMAPs? Why?

Cottage Cheese # 1: Cultured Skim Milk, Cream, Inulin, Salt, Xanthan Gum, Guar Gum, Mono and Diglycerides, Locust Bean Gum, Carageenan, Polysorbate 80, Natural Flavors, Enzymes, Potassium Sorbate and Carbon Dioxide, Vitamin A Palmitate.

Cottage Cheese #2: Ingredients: Cultured Pasteurized Skim Milk, Milk, Maltodextrin, Corn Starch, Salt, Natural Flavor, Lactase Enzyme, Xanthan Gum, Locust Bean Gum, Guar Gum, Vitamin A Palmitate, Sorbic Acid and Carbon Dioxide.

Which of the following pasta sauces is probably lower in FODMAPs? Why?

Pasta Sauce # 1: Italian Plum Tomatoes, Italian Cherry Tomatoes, Italian Olive Oil, Fresh Carrots, Fresh Celery, Fresh Onions, Fresh Garlic, Salt, Fresh Basil. Gluten-free.

Pasta Sauce #2: Tomato Puree, Diced Tomatoes, Extra Virgin Olive Oil, Salt, Spices.

Which of the following jams is probably lower in FODMAPs? Why?

Jam #1: Strawberries, Pure Cane Sugar, Water, Pectin, Lemon Juice Concentrate, Citric Acid.

Jam #2: Water, Strawberries, Maltitol Syrup, Sorbitol, Fruit Pectin, Locust Bean Gum, Natural Flavor, Citric Acid, Potassium Sorbate, Rebiana (Extract from the stevia plant), Calcium Chloride, Red 40.

Which of the following breads is probably lower in FODMAPs? Why?

Bread #1: Filtered Water, Tapioca Starch, Brown Rice Flour, Potato Starch, Sunflower, Oil, Egg Whites, Tapioca Maltodextrin, Evaporated Cane Juice, Brown Rice Syrup or Tapioca Syrup, Yeast, Xanthan Gum, Salt, Baking Powder, Mold Inhibitor (Cultured Corn Syrup, Ascorbic Acid), Ascorbic Acid (Microcrystalline Cellulose and Cornstarch), Enzymes. Gluten free.

Bread #2: Water, Tapioca Starch, Brown Rice Flour, Egg Whites, Resistant Corn Starch, Non-GMO Vegetable Oil (Canola or Sunflower or Safflower), Flax Seed, Cane Syrup, Chia Seed, Yeast, Organic Inulin, Citrus Fiber, Evaporated Cane Juice, Rice Bran, Salt, Pea Protein, Dry Molasses, Gum (Xanthan Gum, Sodium Alginate, Guar Gum, Carageenan, Locust Bean Gum), Sodium Carboxymethyl Cellulose, Cultured Corn Syrup Solids, Enzymes. Gluten free.

Bread # 3: Filtered Water, Tapioca Starch, Brown Rice Flour, Potato Starch, Sunflower Oil, Egg Whites, Evaporated Cane Juice, Tapioca Maltodextrin, Teff Flour, Brown Rice Syrup or Tapioca Syrup, Flax Seed Meal, Yeast, Xanthan Gum, Salt, Baking Powder, Mold Inhibitor (Cultured Corn Syrup, Ascorbic Acid), Dry Molasses, Maltodextrin), Ascorbic Acid (Microcrystalline Cellulose, Cornstarch), Enzymes. Gluten free.

Which of the following snack bars is probably lower in FODMAPs? Why?

Bar #1: Whole Grain Oats, Sugar, Canola Oil, Peanut Butter (Peanuts, Salt), Yellow Corn Flour, Brown Sugar Syrup, Soy Flour, Salt, Soy Lecithin, Baking Soda.

Bar # 2: Organic Rolled Oats, Organic Dried Cane Syrup, Organic Sunflower Oil, Rice Crisp (Rice Flour, Barley Malt Extract, Dried Cane Syrup, Salt, Calcium Carbonate), Honey, Natural Flavors, Organic Barley Flakes, Organic Rye Flakes, Oat Bran, Oat Fiber, Sea Salt, Inulin (Chicory Extract). May Contain Traces of Peanuts, Tree Nuts, Wheat, and Soy. We Source Ingredients That Are Not Genetically Engineered.

Answers and discussion:

Cottage Cheese #2 is probably lower in FODMAPs (Lactaid Cottage Cheese). It contains the enzyme lactase to break down lactose and make it a lactose-free product. The maltodextrin and gums in cottage cheese #2 might have caught your eye, but they are not FODMAPs. Cottage cheese #1 contains an added FODMAP ingredient (inulin) and it is not treated with the lactase enzyme, so it would not be suitable for a low-FODMAP diet.

Pasta Sauce #2 is probably lower in FODMAPs (Cento All-Natural Pasta Sauce). The fact that Pasta Sauce #1 is organic, and that its ingredients are fresh, doesn't matter; it is not suitable for a low-FODMAP diet because it has onion and garlic in it.

Jam #1 is probably lower in FODMAPs (Stonewall Kitchen Strawberry Jam). It is sweetened with cane sugar, which is suitable for a low-FODMAP diet. Strawberries and lemon juice are low in FODMAPs. Pectin is not a FODMAP. Jam #2, on the other hand, is sweetened with two sugar alcohols: maltitol and sorbitol, making it unsuitable for a low-FODMAP diet.

Bread #1 is probably lower in FODMAPs (Udi's White Sandwich Bread). There are no high-FODMAP ingredients in it. Even though it is gluten-free, Bread #2 is not suitable because it has one definite high FODMAP ingredient (inulin) and several ingredients with unknown, but possibly high, FODMAP status (flax seed, citrus fiber, pea protein, dry molasses). Bread #3 is somewhere in between, with no obvious high FODMAP ingredients, but some of unknown status (flax seed meal, and dry molasses). These breads illustrate that you can't just go by the brand name or by the fact that a product is gluten-free. *All three of these are Udi's gluten-free breads, but only one is suitable for a low-FODMAP diet.*

Bar #1 is probably lower in FODMAPs (Nature Valley Crunchy Peanut Butter Granola Bar). Soy flour is the likely FODMAP ingredient, and it is not one of the first ingredients, so is probably present in only a small amount. Although this bar may not be perfect because of the soy flour, it is better than Bar #2, which contains several definite high-FODMAP ingredients, including honey, barley flakes, rye flakes, and inulin. (That Bar #2 is not gluten-free, that it contains traces of wheat or soy, and that it does not contain genetically engineered ingredients are irrelevant facts.)

Why are FODMAPs so Confusing? Data and Discrepancies

The FODMAP concept was originated by researchers at Monash University in Australia, and this group continues to publish most of the emerging FODMAP food composition data. If you live in their part of the world, you might be interested in the excellent low-FODMAP diet material, shopping guides, and cookbooks published by the Eastern Health Clinical School at Monash University. Sales of the Monash University Low FODMAP Diet app help fund ongoing FODMAP research. Books and websites about FODMAPs from a variety of sources are becoming more widely available. Don't misunderstand the difference between published *facts about the FODMAP composition of foods* (for example, how many grams of sorbitol are in an apple) and the *teaching tools* that various medical workers and writers create to communicate whether or not it's OK to eat that apple. Tools might include printable handouts on the internet or at the doctor's or dietitian's office, books like this one, and smartphone apps.

At the heart of each teaching tool is a list of low-FODMAP foods. The Low-FODMAP Pantry and the Label Reading Tips in this book were developed by Patsy Catsos and are based on the available data about the FODMAP content of foods at the time of publication. When people create tools, they make different decisions about which foods to include based on cut-offs for what is considered "high-FODMAP," as well as portion sizes. You can expect some minor variations from one teaching tool and set of recipes to the next. Each tool creator and project team filters the FODMAP data through a different lens, and that's OK. A few minor discrepancies don't diminish the impact of lowering the overall FODMAP load of your diet. In this book, we tend to decide if a food is low in FODMAPs based upon the amount of FODMAPs in a standard serving size, such as ½ cup of vegetables, while another system might shrink the portion down to a very small size if necessary to give the food a "green light." For example, in Patsy's system Brussels sprouts are not in the low-FODMAP pantry. In the Monash University app, which uses a "traffic light" system, they get a green light, but the portion size allowed is very small, only two sprouts. Learning about FODMAPs means learning to live with some conflicting information about which foods you should eat on a low-FODMAP diet.

Look for teaching tools that are written by nutrition professionals who understand the science and who know that high-FODMAP foods aren't "bad foods." If you are using two books or handouts by the same writer, realize that food lists with the later publication date should be more accurate. For example, the food lists in this book are more up-to-date than our previous books. And finally, be patient with us, as we have to revise teaching tools when new facts about FODMAPs are published. As researchers learn more about the FODMAP content of foods, FODMAP status or recommended portions may change.

When new or revised lists of high- and low-FODMAP foods or new tools become available, the inevitable discrepancies can create a little anxiety about whether you've been "doing it right." Our best advice is this: do not let small discrepancies distract you from the big picture. Even with some uncertainties, substantially lowering your overall FODMAP load will help you decide whether FODMAPs are impacting your IBS symptoms and allow you to manage them more effectively.

MEETING YOUR NUTRITION NEEDS

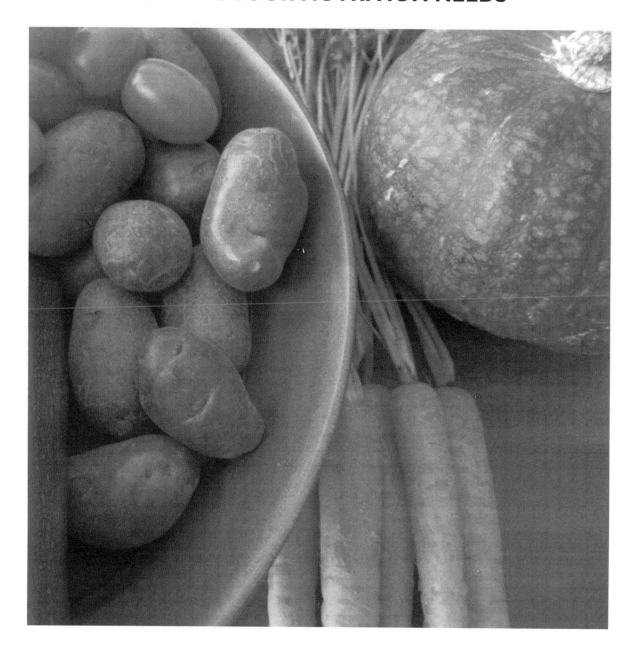

Your nutrient requirements depend on your age, sex, activity level, potential for growth, current weight, and health status. There are so many variables that we can't cover them all in this book. The United States Department of Agriculture (USDA) has an interactive web page you can use to calculate recommended average daily nutrient intake for healthy people. It can be found at http://fnic.nal.usda.gov/fnic/interactiveDRI. Key words to understand here are *calculate*, *average,* and *healthy people*. These calculations are general, estimated targets, not facts about you. No one could achieve the same exact nutrient target every day; for example, people eat more protein some days and less on others, which should average out to the recommendation provided by the calculator. You will note the calculator is designed for health care professionals. That is because goals for nutrient intake often need to be modified if the individual has any medical conditions. For example, many people with IBS or other gastrointestinal conditions would have a very difficult time consuming the number of grams of fiber recommended by this tool, so that goal might have to be adjusted downward. People with documented nutrient deficiencies might need to consume those nutrients in larger amounts than other people until the deficiency is corrected. Also, in our experience, caloric needs are often overestimated using tools like this. In other words, the information from this calculator is just a starting point, and it will give you a rough idea of what you are shooting for. It is important to seek assistance from a dietitian if you have concerns about your (or your child's) weight, growth, or energy needs. Registered dietitian nutritionists are uniquely qualified to evaluate your history and specific circumstances to help you set goals for your nutrient intake.

In the end, people eat foods, not nutrients, so we don't typically encourage our patients to get caught up in calculating how many milligrams of most vitamins or minerals they are consuming. If you choose a wide variety of low-FODMAP foods, your nutrient intake should be just fine. If you choose not to eat certain food groups—for example, if you are a vegan or won't eat your vegetables—you might have more cause for concern, and you should be working with a dietitian who can help you decide what supplements might be in order. Three nutrients deserve special mention because their intake may be at risk on low-FODMAP diets: fiber, protein, and calcium.

Fiber

Use the USDA calculator located at http://fnic.nal.usda.gov/fnic/interactiveDRI to estimate your fiber needs. Remember, these calculations are intended for healthy people. They do not take into account the many medical conditions that can affect the fiber requirements of an individual person, such as IBS, gastroparesis, diverticular disease, Crohn's disease, and ulcerative colitis. Please discuss your individual fiber needs with a health care professional.

Getting enough fiber poses a particular challenge to those on a low-FODMAP diet, because so many high-fiber foods are limited on the diet. Wheat is often our "go to" grain for fiber, in everything from bran flakes to whole-wheat spaghetti. Some of us actually have IBS symptoms because we are choosing too much fiber-fortified food. Breakfast cereals, multi-grain breads, or nutrition bars containing inulin or chicory root may be tolerated by people whose guts function properly, but for people with IBS they contribute to excess gas and bloating because they are so rapidly fermented. So we really have to rethink fiber. There are many ways that scientists have categorized fiber over the years. You might remember references to so-called "soluble fiber" being good for people with IBS, but that isn't relevant here. In the FODMAP world, the most important thing is whether the fiber is rapidly fermentable or not. Suitable fibers for a low-FODMAP diet are not rapidly fermentable. If you tend toward constipation-predominant IBS, and if cutting back on FODMAPs helps reduce gas and bloating but doesn't produce softer or more frequent stools, you may not be eating enough low-FODMAP fiber. Increase your fiber intake *gradually, as tolerated, and not to the point of pain,* by choosing higher-fiber foods more often. Just do the best you can. Portions are given on the following table to accurately communicate the fiber content of these foods, but **only those in bold** must be portion-controlled on the elimination phase of a low-FODMAP diet.

Food/Beverage	Portion	Fiber grams (g)
Brown rice	1 cup prepared	3.5g
Chana dal	**½ cup prepared**	**8g**
Chia seeds	**2 tablespoons**	**5g**
Chick peas, canned, drained	**½ cup**	**5.2g**
Corn pasta	1 cup prepared	6.7g
Cornmeal/polenta, whole grain yellow	1 cup prepared	4.5g
Lentils, canned, drained	**½ cup**	**7.8g**
Low-FODMAP fruits	**½ cup**	**2-3.1g***
Low-FODMAP nuts	**2 tablespoons**	**around 1g**
Low-FODMAP seeds	**2 tablespoons**	**around 2g**
Low-FODMAP vegetables (bold)	**½ cup**	**2-4.4g****
Low-FODMAP vegetables (other)	½ cup cooked	1-3.8g***
Millet	1 cup prepared	2.3g
Millet bread	2 slices (56g)	4g
Oat bran	**1 tablespoon, raw**	**1g**
Oatmeal	**½ cup prepared**	**2g**
Popcorn	2 cups prepared	2.4g
Psyllium husk	**2 tablespoons**	**7g**
Quinoa	1 cup prepared	5.2g
Quinoa/corn pasta	1 cup prepared	4g
Rice bran	1 tablespoon, raw	1.5 g
Sourdough bread, spelt	**2 slices (90g)**	**6g**
Sourdough bread, whole wheat	**2 slices (90g)**	**4g**
White potato, with skin	1 medium	3.6g
White potato, without skin	1 medium	2.3g
Wild rice	1 cup prepared	3g

*Highest fiber choices include wild blueberries, kiwi, oranges, starfruit, papayas
**Highest fiber choices include butternut squash, green beans, turnips, okra
***Highest fiber choices include collard greens, cabbage, spinach, canned tomatoes, carrots, spinach, kale, radishes, summer squash

Protein

Use the USDA calculator located at http://fnic.nal.usda.gov/fnic/interactiveDRI/ to estimate your protein needs. Remember, these calculations are intended for healthy people. They do not take into account the many medical conditions that can raise or lower the protein requirements of individuals, particularly pregnancy, lactation, kidney stones, kidney failure, diabetes, acute illness, and recovery from surgery or trauma. Please discuss your individual protein needs with a health care professional. As a point of reference, adults and teenagers typically need a minimum of 46 grams to 56 grams of protein per day, and often more, depending on body size and all of the factors named above. Plentiful low-FODMAP protein intake is easy for people who eat a variety of animal products. There are no FODMAPs at all in the following good sources of protein, and each 3-ounce serving provides somewhere in the neighborhood of 20-26 grams of protein:

Beef
Buffalo/bison
Chicken
Duck
Lamb
Fish of any kind
Pork
Seafood of any kind
Turkey
Venison

Lacto-ovo vegetarians (vegetarians who eat milk and eggs) and vegans (vegetarians who do not eat milk or eggs) have to work harder at getting enough protein without going overboard on FODMAPs. Nuts, for example, should be consumed only in the recommended portions. Cheese is a source of protein, but by the time you fulfill your protein requirement from cheese you will have consumed more calories than you are likely to need. Powdered peanut butter, such as PB2, has not been analyzed for FODMAPs, but vegans might want to give it a try. Many popular plant-based sources of protein are high in FODMAPs, including veggie burgers and beans. Faux meat products such as prepared tofu sausage and hot dogs are high in FODMAPs because of added garlic and onions. Most of the alternative "milks" are less valuable as sources of protein—check those nutrition fact panels and you will see that a cup of almond or hemp milk beverage usually has 0-3 grams of protein, compared to 8 grams in a cup of lactose-free cow's milk. Soy milk is a decent source of protein; unfortunately, most soy milks sold in the United States are made from whole soybeans and are probably high in FODMAPs; look for 8th Continent brand, which is made from soy protein rather than whole soy beans, and is probably low-FODMAP. Although we aren't huge fans of protein powders, they might be needed at times to help some vegetarians (99% lactose-free whey protein powder, egg white powder, or rice protein powder) and vegans (rice protein powder) meet their protein needs on a low-FODMAP diet. Ambitious vegetarians and vegans can use home-prepared seitan. Seitan is not for people with celiac disease—the main ingredient in seitan is gluten. Because seitan is made from wheat protein (and not the fiber portion of wheat), it is low in FODMAPs when it is made without garlic and onion.

When liberalizing the low-FODMAP diet, vegans must give top priority to good protein sources. If you find your overall capacity to handle FODMAPs is limited, use as much of that capacity as necessary for beans, peas and other proteins. We are going to get into gram amounts for the foods shown below, because minimum protein intakes are not negotiable, and because we want to demonstrate how much more attention it takes to get adequate protein on a vegan diet; plant based-protein sources contain less protein per portion than animal foods. Portions are given to accurately communicate the protein content of these foods, but **only those in bold** must be portion-controlled on the elimination phase of a low-FODMAP diet. These foods can help lacto-ovo-vegetarians and vegans meet their protein needs:

Food/Beverage	Portion	Protein grams (g)
Chana dal	**½ cup prepared**	**5.2g**
Chick peas, canned, drained	**½ cup**	**5.3g**
Corn pasta	1 cup prepared	3.7g
Eggs	1 egg	6.1g
Gluten-free bread	1 slice (25g)	2g
Goat cheese (chèvre)	**1 ounce**	**5.25g**
Hemp milk	1 cup	3g
Lactose-free cottage cheese	½ cup	12g
Lactose-free kefir	1 cup	11g
Lactose-free milk, any % fat	1 cup	8g
Lactose-free yogurt	Small carton (170g)	8g
Lentils, canned, drained	**½ cup**	**9g**
Millet	1 cup prepared	6.1g
Natural cheeses such as Cheddar, Swiss or mozzarella	1 ounce	around 7g
Nuts	**2 tablespoons**	**around 3g**
Peanut or almond butter	**2 tablespoons**	**7g**
Pepitas/pumpkin seeds	**2 tablespoons**	**4.4g**
Protein powders made of 99% lactose-free whey, egg white or brown rice	1 serving	10-20 g (brands vary)
Quinoa	1 cup prepared	8.14g
Quinoa/corn pasta	1 cup prepared	4g
Rice pasta	1 cup prepared	3.1g
Rice, white or brown	1 cup prepared	4.5g
Seitan Breakfast Sausage	1 serving	15.1g
Sourdough bread, white, whole wheat, or spelt	**2 slices (90g)**	**8g**
Soy milk made from soy protein (not whole soy beans)	1 cup	7g
Sunflower seeds	**2 tablespoons**	**3.4g**

Calcium

Recommendations for calcium intake are based on age and don't have to be calculated for each individual based on height, weight, pregnancy, or lactation. When you are comparing your intake to these recommendations, you can count calcium in whole foods, calcium in fortified non-dairy beverages, and calcium in supplements.

Age	Recommended dietary allowance (RDA) for calcium, milligrams (mg) per day
1-3 years old	700mg
4-8 years old	1000mg
9-18 years old	1300mg
19-50 year old women, or 19-70 year old men	1000mg
51-70 year old women	1200mg
71+ year old men and women	1200mg

There are plenty of low-lactose milk products suitable for the elimination phase of the low-FODMAP diet. Unless you have an important personal or medical reason to eliminate them, we recommend you continue to consume cow's milk products. They are major sources of nutrients, especially of calcium, protein, and vitamin D (if they are fortified with vitamin D). Goat's milk has about the same lactose content as cow's milk, and low-lactose versions are not commercially available, so switching to goat's milk won't help you eliminate FODMAPs.

Calcium intake can take a hit if you decide to go "dairy-free" instead of the much easier low-lactose cow's milk route. If you do choose to use almond or hemp milk instead, make sure it is calcium-fortified, and always shake the container before pouring to capture the calcium that has settled to the bottom. And remember that alternative milks fall short on protein. Some people imagine that they will get enough calcium from eating green vegetables or almonds. While these foods do have some calcium, it is but a small fraction of the calcium in a serving of yogurt or kefir, as you can see from the list below. Portions are given to accurately communicate the calcium content of these foods, but **only those in bold** must be portion-controlled on the elimination phase of a low-FODMAP diet:

Food/Beverage	Portion	Calcium (mg)
Almonds	**2 tablespoons**	**36mg**
Calcium-fortified hemp milk or almond milk	1 cup	300mg
Calcium-fortified orange juice	**½ cup**	**175mg**
Canned salmon	¼ cup	221mg
Chia seeds	**2 tablespoons**	**90mg**
Chick peas	**½ cup**	**72mg**
Collard greens	1 cup prepared	357mg
Kale	½ cup cooked	94mg
Lactose-free cottage cheese	½ cup	100mg

Lactose-free kefir	1 cup	300mg
Lactose-free milk, any % fat	1 cup	300mg
Lactose-free yogurt	Small carton (170g)	300mg
Natural cheeses such as cheddar, Swiss or mozzarella	1 ounce	around 200mg
Okra	**½ cup**	**62mg**
Pudding made with lactose-free milk	½ cup	150mg
Rhubarb	**½ cup uncooked**	**133mg**
Sardines	3.75 ounce can	351mg
Sesame seeds	**2 tablespoons**	**176mg**
Soy milk made with soy protein (not whole soy beans)	1 cup	300mg
Spinach	½ cup cooked	123mg
Tempeh	½ cup crumbled	92mg
Tofu, medium, firm or extra-firm	¼ of 14 oz. block	553mg

Reading a food label to determine calcium content can be a little tricky. Rather than telling the consumer how many milligrams of calcium are in one serving of the food, the label states what percent of the "Daily Value" one serving of the food provides. The Daily Value varies for each nutrient; for calcium it happens to be 1000mg. If a food contains 30% of the daily value, it contains 30% of 1000mg, which equals 300mg of calcium. If it contains 35% of the daily value, it contains 350mg of calcium, and so on. A ¼ cup serving of these sardines provides 150mg of calcium.

Nutrition Facts

Serv. Size 1/4 cup (55g)
Servings about 1.5

Calories 120
Fat Cal. 70

* Percent Daily Values (DV) are based on a 2,000 calorie diet.

Amount/serving	%DV*	Amount/serving	%DV*
Total Fat 7g	11%	Total Carb. 0g	0%
Sat. Fat 1.5g	8%	Fiber 0g	0%
Trans Fat 0g		Sugars 0g	
Cholest. 30mg	10%	Protein 13g	
Sodium 130mg	5%		

Vitamin A 0% • Vitamin C 0% • Calcium 15% • Iron 6%

INGREDIENTS: SARDINES, OLIVE OIL, SALT, NATURAL SMOKE FLAVOR.

PLANNING MEALS FOR THE WHOLE FAMILY

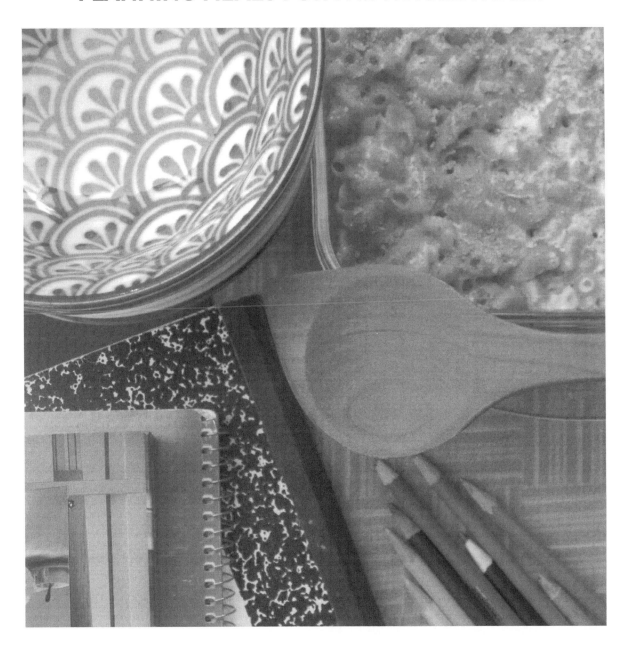

Tips for Menu Planning

Clients often ask for menus they can follow to make following the diet easier. Although the request seems straightforward, it is impossible for one set of menus to get it right for everyone. We all have different priorities and food preferences in mind when we think of a menu that will work for us and our family. A good daily menu should meet nutrient needs, be eye-appealing, have a complementary mixture of textures and spices, be affordable, and use seasonal or available products. You should be able to prepare it in a reasonable amount of time using the kitchen equipment available.

The likelihood of a meal meeting nutrient guidelines is much greater when it includes a good source of protein, a grain or starch (preferably whole grain, for the fiber), a fruit, vegetables (good sources of fiber, vitamins, and minerals), a good calcium source such as milk or yogurt, and a small amount of fat. Sometimes each simply prepared part of the meal will be side-by-side on the plate, other times they will be combined in a recipe. If you skip one of the components at a particular meal, make up for it by choosing a snack to take its place. For example, if you don't drink a glass of lactose-free milk at lunch, make up for it by choosing lactose-free yogurt later, as a snack. If you don't use milk products at all or if you are a vegetarian or vegan, please see Meeting Your Nutrition Needs (page 27) for ideas about substituting alternative sources of protein and calcium.

Dinner	The elements of this well-balanced meal are served separately.
Protein	Grilled chicken
Grain/Starch	Brown rice
Vegetable	Roasted carrots
Fruit	**½ cup fresh pineapple**
Healthy fat	Garlic-infused oil on carrots for roasting
Good calcium source	Glass of lactose-free milk
Good fiber source	(brown rice, carrots, pineapple)

Dinner	Chicken Stir-Fried Rice (recipe). The elements of this (almost) well-balanced meal are combined in the recipe.
Protein	Chicken and eggs (in recipe). Vegetarians substitute tofu
Grain/Starch	Brown rice (in recipe)
Vegetable	Five different vegetables (in recipe)
Fruit	**½ cup fresh pineapple (in recipe)**
Healthy fat	Sesame and garlic-infused oils (in recipe)
Good calcium source	Missing, unless tofu was the source of protein—choose yogurt as a snack some other time during the day
Good fiber source	(brown rice, vegetables, pineapple)

"To snack or not to snack?" is a question you may need to discuss with your health care adviser before menu planning. The right answer depends on your caloric needs for achieving growth or a health body weight, your other health conditions, and your appetite. Gastrointestinal experts note with growing interest that some functions of the small intestine work more efficiently when there is no food in there—in other words, when you are in the "fasting state." People with a "grazing" meal pattern, who eat small amounts continuously throughout the day, are never in the fasting state and may miss out on so-called cleansing waves that keep the population of microbes in the small intestine at healthy levels. This may be especially important for patients who have small intestinal bacterial overgrowth (SIBO). On the other hand, regular meals are important if we expect consistent energy levels and regular functioning of our gastrointestinal tract, so skipping meals is not recommended. Another factor to consider is that large meals typically contain large loads of FODMAPs.

We teach our patients that a consistent meal pattern from one day to the next, with 3-5 hours between moderately-sized meals and snacks, is appropriate for most healthy people and can meet all of these goals. For many people, this would mean three meals plus one or two snacks. Snacks should usually consist of "meal-worthy" foods, not always sweets or salty items. Save those for occasional use unless you need to gain weight. If you have growth concerns or a medical condition besides IBS that impacts your nutrition or food choices, please consult a registered dietitian for assistance with developing an appropriate meal pattern.

How much input should you solicit from other family members while planning menus for your family member's low-FODMAP diet? There is no one right answer here. It will depend on family dynamics and the age of the "patient." Remember, for younger or more anxious children, we recommend you quietly go about your parental business of planning and serving meals that are low in FODMAPs, casually introducing some different brands of condiments and snacks, and developing a sudden interest in making more food from scratch. Family meal-planning experts say you'll get more "buy-in" from family members if they contribute their ideas to meal planning. If you decide this is true for your family, offer younger children a choice between two low-FODMAP foods or recipes. Make sure older family members understand that the basic meal, especially the evening meal, needs to meet the needs of everyone in the family. Luckily, the low-FODMAP recipes in this cookbook taste so good that everyone will be able to enjoy them. Family members who do not have IBS can add high-FODMAP extras served on the side, or at their other meals or snacks.

Here are some more tips that are specific to planning low-FODMAP meals and to this cookbook:

- The easiest plan for a low-FODMAP lunch is to put planned leftovers from the previous night's low-FODMAP dinner in the lunchbox for work or school. Treat yourself to some new bento boxes, microwaveable glass bowls with silicone protective coverings, or insulated thermal containers to make packing lunch easier and more enjoyable.

- A low-FODMAP meal or snack should generally not include more than two servings of **bold** foods so the FODMAP load doesn't get too high. You can make this a little more flexible by using smaller portions. For example, you could have ½ **cup of oatmeal** (1 full bold serving) with **1 tablespoon of walnuts** and ¾ **tablespoon of maple syrup** (half a serving each of two bold items).

- In the meals shown, portions are indicated only for foods that need to be portion controlled because of FODMAPs. Everyone's calorie needs are different. If your calorie needs are smaller, or if you are serving a young child, reduce the portions as needed. If your calorie or protein needs are greater, increase the portions of non-bold foods (or add others) as needed.

- If you don't care for one of the foods suggested, refer to your Low-FODMAP Pantry (page 13) and choose a similar food to replace it.

- Remember that each food or dish named in these meal ideas should be a low-FODMAP version of that food. For example, if "mayonnaise" is listed, it should be a brand that does not contain any high-fructose corn syrup, onions, or garlic. For more brand-name product ideas, visit Patsy at www.pinterest.com/pcatsos, where you can see pictures of products that appear to be suitable for the diet. If you try to purchase any food in the menus ready-made, instead of using our recipes, of course you will be on your own to check the list of ingredients for suitability. For example, take-out fajitas will include lots of onions (high in FODMAPs) compared to the Beef Fajitas recipe in this cookbook.

- Serve water with every meal.

- If you are a coffee or tea drinker, use lactose-free milk or half-and-half rather than regular milk or nondairy creamer; sweeten your beverage with a minimal amount of regular sugar or stevia rather than honey, agave, or sugar-free products.

- Do not eat any food to which you are allergic, even if it appears in these meals.

Key for the meal ideas
Please note the following conventions used throughout the meal ideas: Capitalization: If each word of the food is capitalized, such as Banana Bread, you will find the recipe for that dish in this cookbook.   **Bold:** This food or recipe contains a small amount of FODMAPs. For best results, do not exceed the portion size shown.

Breakfast Ideas

Breakfast 1
1 slice Banana Bread (page 58)
2 tablespoons natural peanut butter
lactose-free cottage cheese

Breakfast 2
½ cup corn flakes
¼ cup strawberries
lactose-free milk
1 tablespoon walnuts

Breakfast 3
1 serving Quinoa Coconut Milk Breakfast Pudding (page 79)
½ banana
lactose-free milk

Breakfast 4
scrambled eggs
bacon
hash browns
½ cup calcium-fortified orange juice

Breakfast 5
1 serving Baked "Pumpkin Pie" Oatmeal (page 76)
lactose-free milk
1 handful pecans

Breakfast 6
½ cup cooked oatmeal
¼ cup raspberries
1 tablespoon walnuts
lactose-free vanilla yogurt

Breakfast 7
1 Carrot Cake Chia Muffin (page 61)
½ cup blueberries
lactose-free raspberry kefir

Breakfast 8 (vegan)
low-FODMAP toast
2 tablespoons almond butter
1 tablespoon strawberry jam
½ banana

Breakfast 9 (vegan)
Seitan Breakfast Sausage (page 78)
hash browns
½ cup calcium-fortified orange juice
1 cup 8th Continent Soymilk

Lunch Ideas

Lunch 1
low-FODMAP sandwich bread
slice cold Turkey Meatloaf (page 105)
lettuce and tomato
½ cup grapes
lactose-free yogurt
1 Chocolate Brownie (page 60)

Lunch 2
Chili Con Quinoa (page 146)
corn chips
½ cup blueberries
lactose-free milk

Lunch 3
rice cakes
2 tablespoons peanut butter
½ banana
red pepper strips
Ranch Dressing (page 128)
lactose-free milk

Lunch 4
low-FODMAP sandwich bread
tuna fish
mayonnaise
lettuce and tomato
½ cup strawberries
lactose-free kefir
potato chips

Lunch 5
mixed salad greens
hard-boiled egg
grilled chicken strips
2 tablespoons balsamic vinegar
olive oil
lactose-free cottage cheese
1 Chocolate Brownie (page 60)

Lunch 6
Mac 'n Cheese with Hidden Squash (page 95)
carrot sticks
½ cup honeydew melon
2 Chewy Chocolate-Chip Cookies (page 62)

Lunch 7
low-FODMAP sandwich bread
turkey breast
provolone cheese
lettuce and tomato
mayonnaise
½ cup blueberries
popcorn

Lunch 8 (vegan)
rice crackers
½ cup Lower-FODMAP Hummus (page 44)
carrot sticks
kiwi

Low-FODMAP breads

Try to find traditionally-made sourdough spelt, white or whole wheat bread in your area; they are the closest low-FODMAP alternative to regular bread (see page 14 and 15 for details). These breads do not contain preservatives, so they have shorter shelf lives and tend to come from local bakeries. Refrigerate or freeze after the first day or two; the bread will still make delicious toast. If sourdough bread isn't available, look for a low-FODMAP bread made of alternative flours such as millet, rice, corn, or tapioca. Some of these breads are marketed as gluten-free and others are not. Gluten-free bread is sometimes suitable for the low-FODMAP diet if other high-FODMAP ingredients have not been added. Alternative breads are usually better when toasted. See www.pinterest.com/pcatsos for product ideas.

Dinner Ideas

Dinner 1
Beef Fajitas (page 85)
baby carrots
Ranch Dressing (page 128)
1 clementine
lactose-free milk

Dinner 2
Baked Salmon with Herbed Cheese Sauce (page 84)
1 serving Roasted Fall Vegetable Salad with Maple Balsamic Vinaigrette (page 116)
½ cup honeydew melon
lactose-free milk

Dinner 3
Mediterranean Chicken on Roasted Potatoes (page 96)
green salad
Lemon Vinaigrette Dressing (page 129)
½ cup cantaloupe
lactose-free milk

Dinner 4
rotisserie chicken from grocery store
buttered rice
1 cup frozen carrots
½ cup fresh pineapple
6 ounces vanilla lactose-free yogurt

Dinner 5
1 serving Fish Tacos with Chipotle Cream (page 89) and Pineapple Salsa (page 88)
1 serving Lime Cabbage Slaw (page 111)
brown rice

Dinner 6
grilled hamburger with **Lisa's Ketchup (page 126)**
baked potato
Ratatouille Casserole (page 102)
1 orange, in wedges

Dinner 7
Turkey Meatloaf (page 105)
Smashed Potatoes (page 118)
1 serving Smoky Kale Salad with Pumpkin Seeds and Shaved Parmesan (page 108)
lactose-free milk

Dinner 8 (vegan)
Oven Roasted Tomato Sauce with Spaghetti and Breadcrumbs (page 87, omit anchovy; use vegan grated "cheese" instead of Parmesan cheese)
Sauteed tofu cubes

Snack Ideas

Snack 1 (vegan)
1 serving Tofu "Almond Joy" Smoothie (page 138)

Snack 2
lactose-free yogurt, **½ cup raspberries, blueberries or strawberries, and 2 tablespoons of walnuts or pecans**

Snack 3
1 Granola Bar (page 137) and a glass of lactose-free milk

Snack 4
1 serving Banana Nut-Butter "Sandwich" (page 135) and a glass of lactose-free milk

Snack 5 (vegan)
1 clementine and **1 handful of almonds**

Snack 6
rice cakes, **2 tablespoons almond or peanut butter,** a glass of lactose-free kefir and **½ cup of grapes**

Snack 7 (vegan)
carrot sticks, a glass of 8th Continent Soymilk

Tips for Grocery Shopping

The process of making a shopping list is just a matter of going through the motions with your meal ideas and your cookbook in hand. This humble weekly task is probably the single most important thing you can do to successfully follow the low-FODMAP diet. It helps to work on your grocery list in the kitchen, so you can easily check your inventory of items on hand; you don't want to over-buy or purchase duplicates. Become a regular at a particular grocery store or farmer's market so you can memorize the layout and where your favorite low-FODMAP foods are located. Write down the items to purchase grouped by department, so you can move efficiently through the store.

Here are some grocery shopping tips that are specific to FODMAPs and to this cookbook:

- Try to choose low-FODMAP fruits, vegetables, and meats that are in season at your grocery store or local farmer's market, which both saves money and ensures you will be purchasing the best quality items.

- Use www.pinterest.com/pcatsos to view pictures of low-FODMAP food products before leaving home, or on your smart phone right at the store. Visual cues really speed up the selection process when you are facing an unfamiliar array of products.

- Check www.shopwell.com, www.fooducate.com, www.foodfacts.com or the web site of your regional supermarket chain to see if product ingredients are listed so you can plan your shopping more carefully at home. Sometimes you can even filter the items on the store web site to show you only products that are available in your own local store. Focus on the list of ingredients on these sites and apps; the rating systems were designed with other considerations in mind and do not relate directly to the low-FODMAP diet.

- Dairy products tend to be regional, so watch for locally available lactose-free brands of which we are not aware.

- Remember that gluten is not a FODMAP. Low-FODMAP foods do not have to be gluten-free. However, some gluten-free foods are suitable for the diet as long as they don't have other high-FODMAP ingredients added, because they don't contain high-FODMAP grains like wheat, barley, and rye. Yes, specialty baked goods and snacks are expensive. You don't have to buy them. Steer around bread, crackers, and pasta and rely on inexpensive low-FODMAP items such as rice, potatoes, and cornmeal for a few weeks.

- Purchase small amount of spices for the recipes in this book from bulk bins at store specializing in natural and organic foods. This costs just pennies compared to the steep prices of herbs and spices in jars.

- If you don't have access to unusual or alternative ingredients in your local market, consider buying online. This is cost-effective for herbs, spices, condiments, and soup stock concentrates in particular, since they don't weigh much. Vitacost.com, Nuts.com, MySpiceSage.com, Penzeys.com, and BobsRedMill.com are some of our favorite sites for purchasing specialty groceries.

- Save yourself some trouble at home by skipping certain items your low-FODMAP family member can't have, and bringing home choices that everyone in the family can enjoy. Why create an opportunity for conflict, when you could just as easily buy grapes instead of apples, plain tortilla chips instead of those seasoned with garlic- and onion, peanuts instead of cashews, or lactose-free ice cream instead of regular?

Sample Low-FODMAP Grocery Standing Order

We suggest that you review the Low-FODMAP Pantry and create your own standing order of items your family enjoys. These will be the items you need on hand at all times to make it easy to follow through on your low-FODMAP diet plans. You can print out your customized list every week and post it in the kitchen. Family members can be taught to circle or write in items that are needed and cross out those that are already on hand in preparation for grocery shopping. Here is a sample that illustrates how laying out the shopping list according to grocery store department can help you shop more efficiently.

Produce	Meat/Fish/Deli	Groceries/Bulk
baby spinach	beef	brown rice cakes
bananas	chicken	brown rice flour
butternut squash	pork chops	canned chick peas
carrots	salmon	canned lentils
cucumber	shrimp	canned tuna
fresh parsley	sweet Italian-style chicken sausage	chocolate chips
grapes	turkey	diced tomatoes
green bell peppers		granulated sugar
kabocha squash		light brown sugar
kale	**Dairy/Eggs/Beverages**	oats
lemons		peanut butter
lettuce	almond milk	peanuts
oranges	cheddar cheese	pecans
potatoes	corn tortillas	potato starch
red bell peppers	eggs	quinoa
scallions	lactose-free cottage cheese	quinoa/corn pasta
spring mix	lactose-free kefir	rice crackers
strawberries	lactose-free milk	rice stick (noodles)
sweet potatoes	lactose-free yogurt	sorghum flour
tofu	Parmesan cheese	tapioca flour
tomatoes	shredded mozzarella cheese	tortilla chips
zucchini		walnuts
		xanthan gum

Condiments	Spices	Frozen Foods
balsamic wine vinegar	allspice	blueberries
Dijon mustard	ancho chile powder	carrots
garlic-infused oil	cinnamon	grated potatoes
mayonnaise	cloves	green beans
soy sauce	coriander	low-FODMAP sandwich bread
	cumin	raspberries
	nutmeg	
	salt	
	smoked paprika	

RECIPE MODIFICATION BASICS

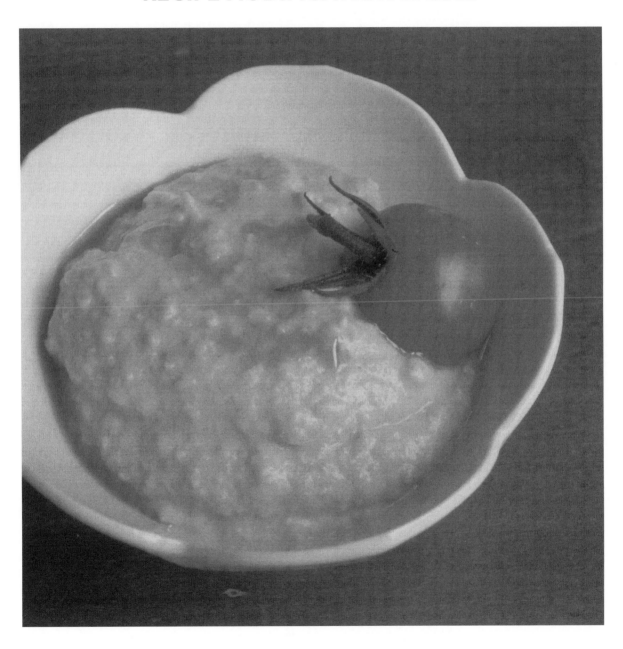

Many of your favorite recipes can be easily adapted for use during a low-FODMAP diet. The first step is to identify high-FODMAP ingredients, and to figure out the function of that ingredient in the original recipe. The high-FODMAP ingredient can sometimes be omitted, a much smaller amount can be used to lower the FODMAP load, or a lower-FODMAP ingredient that serves the same function can be substituted.

One important principle of the FODMAP approach is avoiding large loads of FODMAPs at any one meal or snack. How should you handle a recipe that calls for more than one **bold** ingredient from your pantry? Is such a recipe off limits for the FODMAP elimination diet? Not necessarily. We adjusted the recipes in this book so that eating one serving of the recipe as prepared should still keep you within the guidelines of the elimination diet, and you can do the same when you modify your recipes at home. *Please note: if you choose to eat more than one serving of the recipes in this book, you may be straying above the recommended portion sizes for certain ingredients.*

This Lower-FODMAP Hummus illustrates the thought process for modifying recipes to make them lower in FODMAPs.

Hummus (original recipe)	Lower-FODMAP Hummus
⅔ cup chick peas, dried, uncooked	1 (14.5-ounce) can chick peas, drained and rinsed
¼ cup chick pea cooking water	2 tablespoons water
2 tablespoons fresh lemon juice	4 tablespoons fresh lemon juice
2 tablespoons tahini	2 tablespoons peanut butter
1 tablespoon olive oil	2 tablespoons garlic-infused olive oil
2 cloves garlic	1 teaspoon sesame oil, dark or spicy
½ teaspoon salt	½ teaspoon salt

Starting from the top, use a similar volume of canned, drained chick peas instead of cooking them from scratch; ⅔ of a cup dried chick peas would have yielded about the same amount of chick peas as in a 14.5-ounce can. I've always thought canned chick peas make better hummus anyway, but now we know that a lot of the gassy fiber in chick peas and other legumes leaches out into the canning water during many months of shelf storage and goes down the drain instead of into the hummus. Most hummus recipes call for thinning the hummus with the cooking water or canning water, but this modified recipe uses fresh water and some extra lemon juice and olive oil for thinning to a dipping consistency. We are using peanut butter and sesame oil to reproduce the texture and flavor of tahini, because peanut butter is lower in FODMAPs than tahini. The garlic cloves must go, but we can capture some garlic flavor by using garlic-infused olive oil instead of regular. (Procedure: Measure ingredients into the bowl of a blender or food processor in the order shown. Process until smooth and creamy. Delicious!)

Substitutions for Flavor without FODMAPs

If you lack experience in the kitchen, you may wonder whether recipes will come out right if you change or omit high-FODMAP ingredients. Substitutions might also be necessary if you don't have one an ingredient on hand, or if you have to omit ingredients due to a food allergy or sensitivity. With the exception of baked goods, most recipes will still come out quite well as long as you substitute solids for solids and liquids for liquids. All recipes can have the herbs, spices, and flavorings changed or omitted as needed. Many of the recipes in this book have specific suggestions for substitutions, which we tested for success. Here are a some FODMAP-related substitutions you can try to further modify our recipes or to modify your own conventional recipes as needed.

If the recipe calls for:	Substitute with:	Think about:
Milk	An equal amount of any liquid	The first choice for most people should be lactose-free cow's milk, which is widely available, functions predictably well in recipes, and will make your recipe come out closest to the original in flavor and nutrition. Depending on your caloric needs, you can use skim (non-fat), low-fat, or whole milk. Your choice does not affect the outcome of the recipe technically, though you might prefer the flavor of the whole milk in certain recipes. If you can't drink cow's milk, you can substitute almond milk or hemp milk. In smoothies, you can even use canned coconut milk or coconut cream in place of other fluids if you need to boost calories. These canned coconut products are much more concentrated than other milks, so they shouldn't be used to replace milk in other recipes.
Yogurt or buttermilk	An equal amount of lactose-free yogurt or kefir	If the recipe calls for yogurt or buttermilk, you can substitute an equal amount of lactose-free yogurt or kefir. If you can't purchase ready-made lactose-free yogurt, try our yogurt recipe (page 140). Products that claim to be 99% lactose-free are well-tolerated by most people. In smoothies you can go further than that and substitute any other liquid, such as almond milk or hemp milk. While the texture of the smoothie will certainly change, the smoothie will still be drinkable and tasty.
Onions	Chives, scallions or leek greens PLUS low-FODMAP vegetables as needed to match the original volume of onions	A two-pronged substitution is needed to replace both the flavor and the volume of the onions in the recipe. The flavor of the onions can be provided by the green parts of scallions (green onions), leeks or chives. Or, see pages 122-123 for information about making and using onion-infused oil. An equal amount of a low-FODMAP vegetable can make up for any difference in volume. For example, if a chili recipe calls for 1 cup of chopped onions, you could substitute ¼ cup of scallion greens and ¾ cup of chopped bell peppers or any other combination equaling a total of one cup. A pinch of asafetida, a very strong-smelling Indian spice, adds the right onion flavor notes to certain cooked foods.
Garlic	Garlic-infused oil for an equal amount of the original oil in the recipe	The flavor of garlic is not the problem. You are trying to avoid eating the flesh of the garlic, as well as any of the water-soluble FODMAPs that may leach out into broths or sauces. Garlic powder, garlic salt, and dehydrated garlic are off limits, as well. Substitute garlic-infused oil for some or all of the oil in the original recipe. Or, add garlic-infused oil just for the flavor, even if the original recipe didn't call for oil. You can add a teaspoon or two of garlic-infused oil to almost any vegetable, salad, soup, or stew recipe without any negative impact on the outcome. Or, in recipes calling for sautéed, minced garlic, simply remove the garlic after sautéing it in oil and before adding other ingredients. If you don't care much for garlic in the first place, by all means omit it.

If the recipe calls for:	Substitute with:	Think about:
Honey or agave syrup	Karo light corn syrup (not Karo Lite, which contains sucralose), brown rice syrup or golden syrup	Syrup is both a sweetener and a binder in certain recipes. If the recipe doesn't require much stickiness from the syrup, substitute 100% pure maple syrup. Maple syrup burns easily, though, so watch your food very carefully as it bakes or cooks. You can also substitute sugar as a sweetener in place of honey or agave, but it is a little more complicated because you have to account for the liquid that honey contributes to the recipe. One cup of honey equals approximately 1 ¼ cups sugar plus ¼ cup liquid. Don't try to substitute stevia for the sweetener in baked goods unless using special recipes designed for the purpose. Stevia extract can easily be used to sweeten smoothies and other cold foods. Just add one drop at a time until the desired level of sweetness is achieved.
Pistachios or cashews	An equal amount of walnuts, pecans, almonds or peanuts	All nuts have some FODMAPs, so make sure your portion of even lower-FODMAP nuts stays small, about 2 tablespoons (one small handful).
Pasta, spaghetti, or macaroni	Pasta made from corn, quinoa or rice	Choose a product of similar shape and size. These pastas are often labeled "gluten-free." Although a low-FODMAP diet doesn't have to be gluten-free, many of these products work nicely as long as other high-FODMAP ingredients have not been added.
Flour	For crispy coatings, use Oven-Baked Bread Crumbs, page 130; for thickener, use corn starch	For thickening, use ½ tablespoon of cornstarch or 1 tablespoon of other low-FODMAP flour in place of 1 tablespoon of regular flour. If flour was the main ingredient in a recipe for a cake, bread, biscuit, or cookie recipe, you should choose an alternative recipe that was specifically developed to come out correctly with alternative flours, such as those in this cookbook, developed by Lisa over her 20 years of experience as a wheat-free baker.
Meat, fish or poultry	An equal amount of any other protein source	Use them interchangeably in most recipes. For example, if the recipe calls for a pound of ground pork, you can replace it with an equal amount of ground beef, turkey, or chicken. If the recipe calls for a cup of cooked, diced chicken, you can replace it with a cup of cooked, diced beef, pork, or fish. You can even replace it with a vegetarian form of protein such as a cup of tofu or tempeh if you prefer. Just remember that meat, fish, and poultry shrink about 20% during cooking, so plan accordingly. The quantities of meat, fish, and poultry called for in these recipes are raw, unless otherwise specified. The procedures were designed with extra-lean (90%) ground meats in mind.

THE RECIPES

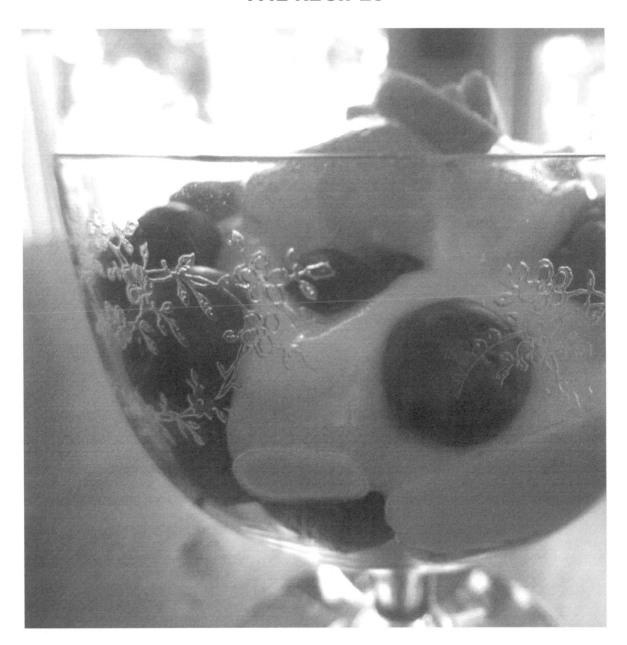

Appetizers

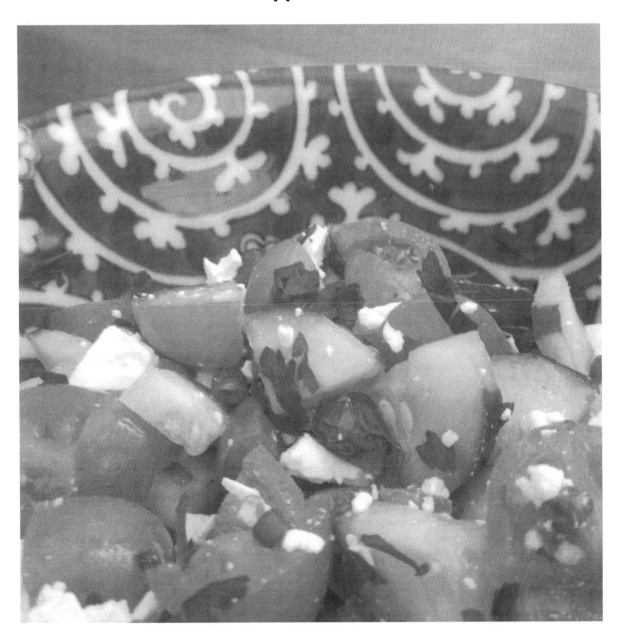

Tomato Feta Salsa

Commercial salsas all contain garlic and onions, but you don't have to go without. This fresh salsa is easy to make and tastes great with tortilla chips!

½ pint grape tomatoes (10-12 tomatoes), diced
    into ¼-inch pieces
1 cup peeled, diced cucumber
1 tablespoon garlic-infused oil
1 scallion, green part only, finely sliced
2 tablespoons minced parsley
⅛ teaspoon salt
¼ cup crumbled feta cheese (1 ounce)
1 teaspoon za'atar (optional)

- Combine all ingredients in a small bowl and allow flavors to blend for 10 minutes.

Servings: 18, 2 tablespoons each

Tips: If cucumbers have thin skins, there is no need to peel them before dicing.

Variations: Dice into larger pieces, add some Lemon Vinaigrette (page 129), and serve as a salad.

Nutrition (per serving): 17 calories, <1g carbohydrates, <1g protein, 1.4g total fat, 45.7mg sodium, <1g fiber, 13.9mg calcium.

Quinoa Falafel with Chick Peas

Falafel is made mostly of chick peas, which are frequently sold as garbanzo beans. This recipe uses a much smaller quantity of chick peas combined with quinoa to make lower-FODMAP patties. These falafels are oven baked, not fried.

1 ½ cups uncooked quinoa, rinsed
¾ teaspoon salt
1 cup canned chick peas, rinsed, drained
1 tablespoon ground cumin
1 ½ teaspoons ground coriander
½ cup finely minced parsley
2 scallions, green part only, finely minced
½ teaspoon baking soda
¼ teaspoon ground black pepper
2 tablespoons garlic-infused oil
2 large eggs, lightly beaten
2 tablespoons canola oil

- Preheat oven to 425° F. Coat two baking pans each with 1 tablespoon canola oil.
- Combine quinoa, 2 ¾ cups water, and salt in a covered saucepan and bring to a boil. Turn heat down and simmer until all water is absorbed, 12-14 minutes. Remove from heat and let sit for 5 minutes. Mash chick peas in a large mixing bowl. Mix in cooked quinoa, cumin, coriander, parsley, scallion greens, baking soda, pepper, and garlic-infused oil. Stir in eggs until combined.
- Coat a ⅓-cup measure with baking spray or oil and pack quinoa mixture into cup. Unmold falafel onto baking pan. Press down lightly with your hand to flatten to ½-inch thickness. Bake in lower third of the oven until golden brown and crispy, 16-18 minutes. Remove from oven, coat tops lightly with baking spray or oil, and turn falafels over. Bake until golden brown on the other side, about 10 minutes. Serve hot, topped with Tomato Feta Salsa (page 50).

Servings: 7 servings, 2 falafels each

Tips: Use canned, rinsed chick peas which are lower in FODMAPs than freshly cooked chick peas.

Nutrition (per serving): 272 calories, 32.3g carbohydrates, 9g protein, 12.2g total fat, 467.6mg sodium, 4.6g fiber, 54.9mg calcium.

Arepas with Basil, Tomatoes, and Mozzarella

Kids will enjoy making this easy recipe because the dough feels like clay. Arepas are often split open and stuffed with filling. Here they are made smaller, left whole, and served with a tasty, simple topping. Use this recipe as a starting point to create your own combinations. Arepa flour comes in yellow and white and is found in the Latin section of supermarkets. It is a specially prepared, precooked corn meal often labeled "masarepa, harina precocida." The package may also list "harina de maiz refinada precocida" (refined, precooked corn flour). Several name brands are Harina PAN, Doñarepa, Areparina, Harina Juana, and Goya. Regular cornmeal, or "masa harina" (flour for tacos), will not work – arepas will crumble.

Topping:
4 ounces mozzarella cheese, diced into small
    cubes
2 medium tomatoes (10 ounces total), diced into
    ¼-inch pieces
2 tablespoons garlic-infused oil
10 fresh basil leaves, sliced
⅛ teaspoon salt
Several generous grinds of black pepper

Arepas:
2 cups arepa flour (masarepa), yellow or white
1 teaspoon salt
3 cups boiling water
2 tablespoons extra virgin olive oil
2 tablespoons canola oil (for frying)

- Preheat oven to 400° F.
- Stir topping ingredients together in a small bowl and allow flavors to blend for a few minutes.
- Combine arepa flour and salt in a large bowl. Add 2 ½ cups boiled water and the olive oil, and mix until a dough forms that is like slightly sticky child's play dough. Knead the dough a few times then let it rest for 5 minutes. Form a piece of dough into a test 1 ½" ball and flatten with your hand. If dough crumbles or falls apart (a few cracks along edges are fine), return to the bowl and knead in more water a tablespoon or two at a time. Alternatively, if dough is too wet and sticky, knead in more flour a tablespoon or two at a time. Let dough rest 5 minutes.
- Form 24 1 ½-inch balls. Use the bottom of a dinner plate or pan to press down and flatten ball into a circle 2-inch wide and ¼-inch thick. Smooth dough edge with fingers where it may crack slightly. To speed up process, space 2-3 balls several inches apart and press all of them at once.
- Heat a large skillet on medium-high heat until hot. Coat pan with baking spray and add 1 tablespoon of canola oil. Add half of the arepas, cover pan, and cook without moving until a medium-dark brown crust forms, 5 to 7 minutes. Coat uncooked side of arepas with baking spray or oil, turn over, and cook uncovered to brown on the other side, spraying pan with additional baking spray. Keep arepas warm in oven.
- Spoon topping over the arepas and serve warm.

Servings: 12, 2 arepas each

Tips: To divide dough evenly into twenty-four balls, form dough into a large pie-shaped loaf. Cut into 6 wedges, then cut each wedge into 4 more wedges. Roll each piece into a 1 ½-inch ball. Leftover arepas can be refrigerated and reheated in a 350° F. oven or microwave. Arepas without topping can be frozen.

Substitutions: Use feta cheese or grated Parmesan instead of mozzarella.

Variations: Try adding ½ cup shredded Parmesan cheese to arepa flour. For a melted cheese version, make the tomato topping without mozzarella. Top each cooked arepa with a small piece of mozzarella and broil until cheese melts. Top with the chopped tomato and basil mixture.

Nutrition (per serving): 93 calories, 11g carbohydrates, 2.2g protein, 4.4g total fat, 140.5mg sodium, <1g fiber, 39.6mg calcium.

Spiced Carrot Dip

Roasted carrots with toasted spices make a surprisingly exotic dip. This dip tastes great on sandwiches and burgers.

1 pound carrots, peeled
3 tablespoons garlic-infused oil, divided
½ teaspoon coriander
½ teaspoon cumin
½ teaspoon smoked paprika
⅛ teaspoon salt, plus a little more for sprinkling
    on carrots
Several grinds black pepper
½ teaspoon lemon zest
1 tablespoon lemon juice
⅛ teaspoon cayenne pepper (optional)
⅓ cup plain lactose-free yogurt

Tips: No food processor or blender? Mash carrots with a potato masher or pastry blender.

Substitutions: If you don't eat dairy, you can leave out the yogurt. Add 1 tablespoon additional oil.

Nutrition (per serving): 47 calories, 4.1g carbohydrates, <1g protein, 3.3g total fat, 51.1mg sodium, 1.1g fiber, 24.9mg calcium.

- Preheat oven to 425° F. Coat a baking sheet with baking spray or oil. Cut carrots into similar sized pieces about 3-inches long by ½-inch thick and place on the baking sheet. Drizzle with 1 tablespoon oil and sprinkle with salt. Roast in the bottom third of the oven until browned, 12-15 minutes. Turn pieces and roast until soft, 5-7 minutes more. Remove from oven.
- While carrots are roasting, add remaining 2 tablespoons garlic-infused oil, coriander, cumin, smoked paprika, and salt to a small skillet on medium heat. Stir until fragrant, about 2 minutes, and remove from heat. Transfer roasted carrots into a food processor and add black pepper, lemon juice, zest, and cayenne. Pulse into a chunky puree. Add yogurt and pulse to mix. With processor running, drizzle in spices and oil until carrots turn into a thick, spreadable dip. Adjust taste with salt, pepper, and lemon juice.

Servings: 13, 2 tablespoons each

Zucchini Quinoa Fritters

This is a great recipe for encouraging kids to eat their vegetables. Serve as an appetizer, side, or light meal. Serve fritters with a spoonful of Oven-Roasted Tomato Sauce (page 87), Romesco Sauce (page 98), Arugula Spinach Pesto (page 127), or 10-Minute Salsa (page 130).

4 medium zucchini (about 2 pounds)
1 cup water
1 ¼ teaspoons salt, divided
½ cup uncooked quinoa, rinsed
⅓ cup of sliced scallions, green part only
¼ cup minced fresh dill or parsley
1 teaspoon lemon zest (optional)
¼ teaspoon ground black pepper
½ cup grated Parmesan (2 ounces)
2 large eggs
½ cup Low-FODMAP All-Purpose Flour (page
    57)
2 tablespoons canola oil for frying
Sour cream (optional)

Tips: Leftover fritters may be frozen and reheated on a baking sheet at 350° F until crisp.

Substitutions: Brown rice flour can be used instead of Low-FODMAP All-Purpose Flour. Yellow summer squash can be used in place of zucchini, or use a combination. Romano, cheddar, or Gouda can be used in place of Parmesan. One teaspoon dried basil and ½ teaspoon dried oregano can be used in place of fresh herbs.

Variations: For a Mexican version, replace dill and lemon zest with ¼ cup chopped cilantro leaves. Replace Parmesan with cheddar. Add 2

- Grate zucchini on the large holes of a box grater and place in a colander in the sink. Sprinkle 1 teaspoon salt evenly over zucchini and let sit for 20 minutes, mixing a few times.
- Measure 1 cup water, ¼ teaspoon salt and quinoa into a 1-quart saucepan, cover and bring to a boil. Turn down heat to a simmer and

cook until water is absorbed and the yellow tail of the grain emerges, 10-12 minutes. Remove from heat and let sit covered for 5 minutes.
- Squeeze water out of the zucchini with your hands and place it in a large mixing bowl, repeating until all the zucchini is drained. Stir in scallion greens, dill, lemon zest, and grated cheese.
- Beat eggs in a small bowl. Pour eggs over vegetables and stir until combined. Sprinkle flour evenly over fritter mixture while stirring.
- Coat a large skillet on medium-high heat with baking spray and add 2 teaspoons of oil. When oil shimmers, use a ¼-cup measure to scoop batter into the skillet and spread to form 4-inch rounds. Fry until dark golden brown, turn over and fry on the other side, 3-4 minutes per side. For each batch, repeat spraying pan and adding 2 teaspoons of oil. Place cooked fritters on a baking sheet in a 200° F oven to keep warm. Serve with a dollop (2 teaspoons per fritter) of sour cream.

Servings: 10, 2 fritters each

teaspoons Chili Powder Mix (page 125). For an Italian version, omit dill, add 1 teaspoon dried basil, ½ teaspoon dried oregano, and ¼ cup parsley.

Nutrition (per serving): 135 calories, 15.2g carbohydrates, 6.2g protein, 6.1g total fat, 394.4mg sodium, 2.2g fiber, 103.6mg calcium.

Thai Sweet and Salty Pork in Lettuce Wraps

This quick, light dish, often served as an appetizer, can be eaten as a meal on a hot day as it requires minimal cooking. Kids particularly like this meal, which is eaten out of hand.

1 head leaf lettuce (Boston, butter, red, or green leaf)
1 cucumber, peeled
1 red bell pepper, seeded and cut into thin strips
2 peeled carrots, shredded or cut into thin rounds
½ cup fresh mint leaves
¼ cup fresh cilantro leaves
2 clementines or tangerines, peeled and sectioned
1 tablespoon peeled, finely minced ginger root
1 pound extra-lean ground pork
2 teaspoons garlic-infused oil
3 tablespoons fish sauce
¼ cup packed light brown sugar
4 scallions, green part only, sliced
¼ teaspoon ground black pepper
½ teaspoon red pepper flakes (optional)
½ cup roasted salted peanuts, coarsely chopped
2 cups cooked brown or white rice, room temperature

- Separate each lettuce leaf from the head, keeping leaves whole. Wash and spin dry. Slice cucumber into thin half rounds. Place the vegetables, herbs, and orange sections on a large serving platter
- Heat oil in a large skillet on medium-high heat and add ginger root. Stir for 45 seconds. Add pork and stir, breaking up meat until it is browned and crumbled. Add fish sauce, brown sugar, scallion greens, black pepper, and chili flakes. Stir until liquid has evaporated, 4-5 minutes. Remove from heat, stir in chopped peanuts, and place in a serving bowl.
- To serve: Each person places a whole lettuce leaf on a plate. Top with 2 tablespoons meat filling, 2 tablespoons rice, a few slices of cucumber, bell pepper, carrots, mint leaves, and cilantro leaves. Top with orange section. Fold the leaf edges over to enclose the filling and enjoy.

Servings: 8

Tips: If cucumber is thin-skinned, it needn't be peeled. Choose a fish sauce with 700mg of sodium or less per tablespoon such as Tiparos brand, available at Asian markets. If you aren't able to buy at least 90% lean pork, turkey, or chicken, drain excess fat after browning meat and before proceeding with the recipe.

Substitutions: Soy sauce may be substituted for fish sauce if necessary. Fresh pineapple chunks or halved navel orange sections can be used in place of clementines. Asian rice vermicelli, cut into 3-inch lengths, can be used in place of rice.

Variations: Ground turkey or chicken can be used instead of ground pork. Fill endive leaves with pork and top with a clementine section, mint, and cilantro (omit rice). Or, serve on top of rice crackers.

Nutrition (per serving): 258 calories, 32.9g carbohydrates, 18.2g protein, 6.7g total fat, 354.6mg sodium, 4.4g fiber, 66mg calcium.

Baking and Desserts

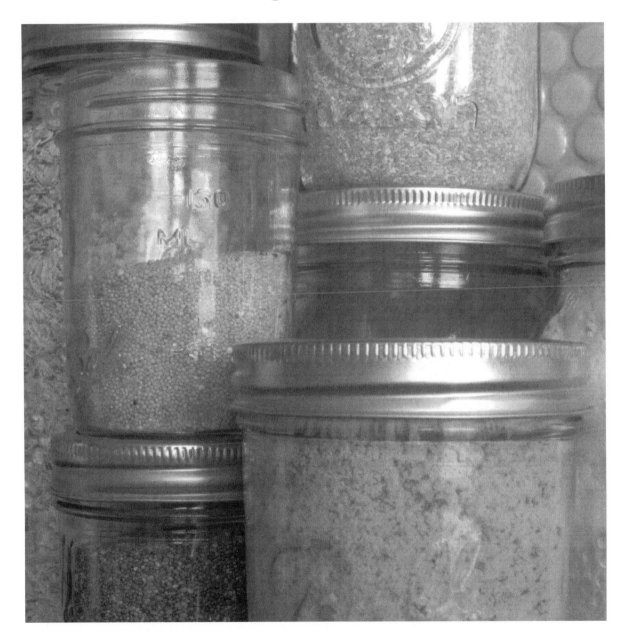

Any discussion of low-FODMAP baking must start with the subject of flour. Ordinary all-purpose flours, cake flours, bread flours and whole wheat flours are made from wheat. Wheat is a high-FODMAP cereal grain, and all of the flours made from it are high in FODMAPs. Therefore, low-FODMAP baking must use flours from alternative grains. No single alternative flour can replicate the unique starch and protein composition of wheat flour. Combinations of these flours must be used to make the best baked goods. Low-FODMAP flour blends and recipes have their roots in gluten-free baking, though gluten itself is not a FODMAP.

Note that certain foods and ingredients made from wheat are low-FODMAP due to processing, for example wheat starch or traditionally made sourdough breads (see page 14 for more about sourdough breads).

Low-FODMAP Baking Mix

After 25 years of tinkering with commercial and homemade baking mixes, Lisa believes that this versatile whole grain, low-FODMAP baking mix makes excellent baked goods with texture and taste similar to wheat flour recipes. It is also higher in nutrition and fiber than most commercial alternative baking mixes. Because the baking mix already contains sugar, leavener (rising agent), salt, and xanthan gum, you only need to add a few additional ingredients and most recipes will be in the oven in 10 minutes or less.

1 cup brown rice flour
1 cup light sorghum flour
1 cup oat flour (3.25 ounces)
½ cup tapioca starch/flour
½ cup potato starch
2 tablespoons aluminum-free baking powder
⅓ cup granulated sugar
1 teaspoon salt
2 teaspoons xanthan gum

- Combine ingredients in an airtight container and shake to mix well. Shake or stir the mix every time before measuring.

Yield: 4 ½ cups

"People with gluten-related disorders should use certified gluten-free oats to make oat flour. Others can use regular commercial oats."

Tips: To make 1 cup of oat flour, grind 1 cup plus 2 tablespoons old fashioned rolled oats in a blender, food processor, or clean coffee mill until a flour texture is reached. If you bake frequently, why not double the recipe? It keeps well in an airtight container.

Substitutions: 1 cup minus 2 tablespoons of commercially ground oat flour can be used in place of home-ground oat flour. Cornstarch can be used in place of potato starch.

Nutrition (entire recipe): 2208 calories, 480.3g carbohydrates, 41.7g protein, 18.1g total fat, 5505.6mg sodium, 31.5g fiber, 1750.5mg calcium.

Low-FODMAP All-Purpose Flour

This flour mix replaces wheat flour cup-for-cup in recipes. This is a mixture of flours only and does not contain any leaveners or binders. It makes baked goods with a fine crumb. Do not confuse with Low-FODMAP *Baking Mix* (previous page) which is a ready-to-bake mix and contains sugar, leaveners, and xanthan gum and is used for baked goods with a larger crumb.

> 1 ½ cups brown rice flour
> 1 ½ cups white/light sorghum flour
> 1 cup tapioca starch/flour
> 1 cup potato starch

Nutrition (entire recipe): 2487 calories, 558.8g carbohydrates, 42.5g protein, 13.1g total fat, 114.2mg sodium, 32.3g fiber, 130.1mg calcium.

- Mix all ingredients together in a large airtight container. Keeps at room temperature for up to 4-8 weeks, or longer in the refrigerator or freezer. Mix flour every time before measuring.

Yield: 5 cups

Almond Blueberry Muffins

Grinding whole almonds to make your own almond flour is easy. Chia seeds improve the texture and add fiber.

> ⅔ cup whole, toasted almonds
> ½ cup packed light brown sugar
> 3 tablespoons ground chia seeds
> 1 ½ cups Low-FODMAP Baking Mix (previous page)
> 2 large eggs
> ¼ cup oil
> 1 ¼ cups lactose-free milk
> 1 teaspoon vanilla extract
> ¾ teaspoon almond extract
> 1 ¼ cups frozen wild blueberries or 1 ½ cups large fresh blueberries
> Coarse, raw sugar, for sprinkling on top (optional)

Tips: If using frozen berries, there is no need to thaw them. Microwave frozen muffins for 30-45 seconds to thaw.

Substitutions: Almond milk or hemp milk can be used in place of lactose-free milk. Two tablespoons of whole chia seeds can be used in place of 3 tablespoons ground chia seeds; reduce milk to 1 cup plus 1 tablespoon.

Time savers: Almonds can be purchased already ground into almond flour/meal. ⅔ cup whole almonds equals 1 cup minus 2 tablespoons of almond flour/meal.

Nutrition (per serving): 228 calories, 27.1g carbohydrates, 7.2g protein, 10.8g total fat, 220mg sodium, 2.8g fiber, 99.5mg calcium

- Preheat oven to 375° F. Coat a 12-cup muffin pan with baking spray or oil.
- Pulse almonds and brown sugar together in a food processor until mixture looks like fine breadcrumbs. Add chia seeds and baking mix and pulse to mix.
- Beat eggs in a large mixing bowl. Add oil, milk, and extracts and whisk. Pour dry ingredients into wet, stir until combined, and let batter sit 5 minutes. It will look like a thick cake batter. If too thick, add a few tablespoons of milk. Stir in blueberries.
- Divide batter into muffin cups. They will be nearly full. Sprinkle with coarse sugar. Bake until a toothpick inserted comes out clean, 20-23 minutes.
- Cool 15 minutes. Run a knife around muffin cup edges to loosen, and remove them to a baking rack to cool. Do not cool them in the pan or they will become soggy. Muffins keep 24 hours unrefrigerated. Refrigerate or freeze for extended storage.

Servings: 12

Banana Bread

This classic, moist banana bread tastes great as a snack with tea, or spread with almond butter for breakfast.

1 ¾ cups Low-FODMAP Baking Mix (page 56)
½ teaspoon baking soda
1 teaspoon cinnamon
¼ teaspoon grated nutmeg
½ teaspoon allspice (optional)
2 large eggs
⅓ cup canola oil
½ cup packed light brown sugar
3 tablespoons chia seeds
1 ½ cups mashed ripe banana (3-4 bananas)
½ cup lactose-free milk
2 teaspoons vanilla
½ cup coarsely chopped pecans or walnuts

- Preheat oven to 350° F. Lightly coat a loaf pan with baking spray or oil.
- In a small bowl, mix together Low-FODMAP Baking Mix, baking soda, cinnamon, nutmeg, and allspice.
- Beat the eggs in a large mixing bowl. Stir in oil, brown sugar, bananas, chia seeds, and vanilla until blended. Add flour mixture to the wet ingredients and mix until no streaks of flour remain. Fold in nuts.
- Pour batter into the prepared loaf pan (it will be very full). Bake for 55-60 minutes or until a toothpick inserted in the center comes out clean. Cool in pan for 20 minutes, then remove banana bread from pan to a cooling rack to prevent the bread from becoming soggy. Refrigerate or freeze for extended storage.

Servings: 12

Tips: Too many ripe bananas? Peel and break each one in half and freeze in a zip-top bag; two pieces equals one banana. Later, defrost in a microwave, or place bananas in a zip-top bag, squeeze air out, and immerse bag in a bowl of hot water.

Variations: For muffins, coat 12-14 muffin cups with baking spray or oil. Fill muffin cups ¾ full. Bake 15-18 minutes or until toothpick inserted comes out clean.

Substitutions: Omit chia seeds and add ¼ cup more baking mix.

Nutrition (per serving): 269 calories, 35.2g carbohydrates, 4.6g protein, 13.2g total fat, 247mg sodium, 5g fiber, 131.5mg calcium.

Berry Parfait with Lemon Crème

This light and easy dessert tastes similar to lemon cheesecake, and is pictured on our book cover.

1 cup lactose-free cottage cheese
1 tablespoon plus 2 teaspoons fresh lemon juice
1 ½ teaspoons lemon zest
⅓ cup confectioners' sugar
½ teaspoon vanilla extract
1 ½ cup sliced strawberries, blueberries, and
    raspberries, mixed
3 tablespoons coarsely chopped, toasted almonds

- Measure cottage cheese, lemon juice, zest, confectioners' sugar, and vanilla into blender. Blend mixture until smooth and creamy, 1-2 minutes. Lemon crème can be used right away or chilled 1 hour for a thicker texture.
- Place ¼ cup of fruit in each of 3 wine glasses. Top each with about 3 tablespoons of lemon crème. Divide remaining fruit among the glasses and top each with remaining lemon crème. Sprinkle each parfait with chopped almonds.

Servings: 3

Substitutions: ¼ cup granulated sugar can be used in place of ⅓ cup confectioners' sugar. If using granulated sugar, process sugar in the blender first for 1 minute before adding other ingredients

Time savers: Replace chopped almonds with 1 tablespoon toasted coconut flakes or gluten-free cookie crumbs (gingersnap, shortbread, or animal crackers).

Nutrition (per serving): 201 calories, 27.6g carbohydrates, 11.8g protein, 5.5g total fat, 167.5mg sodium, 3.1g fiber, 77.4mg calcium.

Very Berry Crisp

This fruit crisp can be made with 10 cups of any combination of berries except blackberries, which are high in FODMAPs.

½ cup granulated sugar
2 tablespoons cornstarch
Zest from one lemon
4 cups sliced strawberries
4 cups wild blueberries
2 cups raspberries
1 tablespoon fresh lemon juice
2 cups uncooked old fashioned oats
⅔ cup Low-FODMAP All-Purpose Flour (page 57)
1 cup packed light brown sugar (or 1 cup granulated sugar)
½ teaspoon cinnamon
½ teaspoon salt
1 stick (½ cup) unsalted butter
1 teaspoon vanilla

- Preheat oven to 350° F. Lightly coat a 9 x 13-inch baking pan with baking spray or oil.
- In a large bowl, mix together sugar, cornstarch and zest. Add berries and lemon juice, and gently stir. Pour berries into baking pan.
- Combine oats, flour, sugar, cinnamon, and salt in a medium bowl. Melt butter, then stir in vanilla extract. Pour melted butter over oat mixture and stir until crumbly. Sprinkle topping evenly over berries and bake until bubbling and golden brown, 45-55 min.

Servings: 12

Tips: If you are using frozen berries, place them in a bowl and cover with warm water until thawed; drain fruit before proceeding. If berries are very tart, use up to ⅔ cup sugar.

Substitutions: Substitute up to 4 cups of rhubarb for part of the berries; add an extra ⅓ to ½ cup of sugar and 1 more teaspoon of cornstarch when using rhubarb.

Variations: For an almond topping, use ½ cup almond meal/flour plus 3 tablespoons Low-FODMAP All-Purpose Flour instead of ⅔ cup Low-FODMAP All-Purpose Flour. Add ½ teaspoon almond extract to the melted butter in addition to vanilla.

Time savers: Halve recipe and bake in an 8 x 8-inch baking pan for 30-35 minutes.

Nutrition (per serving): 354 calories, 62.1g carbohydrates, 6g protein, 10.1g total fat, 107.8mg sodium, 8g fiber, 59.8mg calcium.

Chocolate Fruit and Cookie Dip

Serve this creamy treat as a dip for strawberries, bananas, or low-FODMAP cookies. Though it takes just minutes to make, plan ahead as it is best served chilled.

¼ cup plus 1 tablespoon granulated sugar
1 cup lactose-free cottage cheese
3 tablespoons unsweetened cocoa powder
½ teaspoon vanilla
1 pint strawberries, washed and hulled (¾ pound)
1 banana, peeled, cut into ½-inch thick rounds
Low-FODMAP versions of cookies such as gingersnaps, butter cookies, or animal crackers (optional)

- Grind sugar in the blender until fine, 30-60 seconds. Add cottage cheese, cocoa powder, and vanilla and blend until smooth, scraping down sides once, about 1 minute. Pour into a serving dish and chill, 45-60 minutes. Chill in the freezer for faster results.

Servings: 6

Tips: Freeze for 2-3 hours for a lactose-free, ice cream-like dessert.

Substitutions: ⅓ cup plus 3 tablespoons of confectioners' sugar can be used in place of granulated sugar. Omit grinding.

Nutrition (per serving): 169 calories, 36.4g carbohydrates, 6.4g protein, 1.2g total fat, 85.4mg sodium, 4.4g fiber, 46.5mg calcium.

Chocolate Brownies

These brownies are rich even without the glaze, so you can decide just how decadent you want them to be.

½ cup plus 1 tablespoon unsweetened cocoa
    powder, divided
¾ cup plus 1 tablespoon Low-FODMAP All-
    Purpose Flour (page 57), divided
½ teaspoon baking powder
¼ teaspoon salt
¼ teaspoon xanthan gum
1 stick unsalted butter (¼ pound), melted
1 ¼ cup packed light brown sugar
3 eggs
2 teaspoons vanilla
½ cup semi-sweet chocolate morsels
½ cup chopped pecans, hazelnuts, almonds, or
    walnuts (optional)

Variations: Add 1 teaspoon instant coffee granules to the batter with the cocoa powder to intensify the chocolate flavor.

Nutrition (per serving): 168 calories, 22.2g carbohydrates, 2.2g protein, 9g total fat, 60.3mg sodium, 1.6g fiber, 30.9mg calcium.

- Preheat oven to 350° F. Coat the bottom and sides of a 9 x 9-inch pan with baking spray or oil.
- Mix 1 tablespoon cocoa powder and 1 tablespoon Low-FODMAP All-Purpose Flour in a small bowl. Pour the mixture into the center of the oiled pan, and tilt to coat bottom and sides. Tap out excess.
- In a small bowl combine ½ cup cocoa powder, ¾ cup Low-FODMAP All-Purpose Flour, baking powder, salt, and xanthan gum.
- Beat melted butter and sugar in a large bowl on medium speed 1-2 minutes. Add eggs one at a time, beating until smooth. Add vanilla and flour mixture and beat until smooth. Fold in chocolate morsels and chopped nuts.
- Pour batter into pan and spread evenly, rapping pan on the counter. Bake until a toothpick inserted in center comes out clean, 25-30 minutes. When brownies are cool, run a knife around the edges of the pan. Turn pan upside down on a plate and firmly rap on the bottom of the pan to release brownies in one piece. Place a cutting board over brownies, turn over, and remove the plate. Brownies are now right side up. If adding Chocolate Glaze, frost 30 minutes before cutting.

Servings: 20

Mocha Glaze

1 cup confectioners' sugar
3 tablespoons unsweetened cocoa powder
3-4 tablespoons lactose-free milk
½ teaspoon vanilla
¼ teaspoon instant coffee granules
2 tablespoons butter, cut into small pieces

Nutrition (per serving): 14 calories, <1g carbohydrates, <1g protein, 1.3g total fat, 15.8mg sodium, <1g fiber, 4.1mg calcium.

- Whisk together confectioners' sugar and cocoa in a small bowl.
- In a separate, small microwave safe bowl, heat remaining ingredients until butter melts. Stir to dissolve coffee, then add cocoa mixture and stir until glaze is smooth and pourable, adding more milk a teaspoon at a time if needed. Pour warm glaze evenly over the brownies and use an offset spatula to quickly spread glaze over the top.

Servings: 20

Carrot Cake Chia Muffins

Chia seeds add crunch, fiber, and nutrition to these moist muffins, and replace a large amount of oil in the recipe. If you don't like the chia seed texture, grind them in a coffee grinder or blender. A Carrot Cake Chia Muffin is pictured on the cover of this cookbook.

¼ cup whole chia seeds
1 cup lactose-free milk
2 ¼ cups Low-FODMAP Baking Mix (page 56)
⅔ cup packed light brown sugar
¼ teaspoon baking soda
1 ½ teaspoon ground cinnamon
¼ teaspoon ground ginger
¼ teaspoon ground nutmeg
⅛ teaspoon ground cloves
2 large eggs
⅓ cup canola oil
1 ½ teaspoons vanilla
1 ½ cups packed, finely grated carrots (about 2
    large, or 5-6 ounces)
½ cup coarsely chopped pecans or walnuts
    (optional)
Raw sugar crystals (optional)

Nutrition (per serving): 276 calories, 37.6g carbohydrates, 4.8g protein, 12.7g total fat, 290.2mg sodium, 4.2g fiber, 154.4mg calcium.

- Preheat oven to 400° F. Place oven rack slightly above the middle rack position. Coat a 12-cup muffin pan with baking spray or oil.
- Whisk chia seeds and 1 cup milk together in a medium bowl and set aside for 3-4 minutes. Seeds will turn gel-like in a few minutes.
- Stir Low-FODMAP Baking Mix, brown sugar, baking soda, cinnamon, ginger, nutmeg, and cloves together in a small bowl until no lumps of sugar remain.
- Add eggs to the milk and chia mixture and whisk until well blended. Mix in oil and vanilla. Stir flour mixture into the liquid ingredients until a thick, spoonable wet batter forms. Add more milk if needed. Fold in carrot and nuts.
- Pour batter into muffin cups until nearly full. Sprinkle with raw sugar. Bake until a toothpick inserted in the middle comes out clean, 16-18 minutes. Cool muffins for 20 minutes. Run a knife around muffin cups and remove muffins to a baking rack to cool completely to prevent them from becoming soggy.

Servings: 12

Why do some recipes call for aluminum-free baking powder but others do not?
Alternative flours can be heavier than regular flour, so more baking powder is often needed. Although ordinary baking powders will provide adequate leavening in larger amounts, some people can detect a metallic taste. So our Low-FODMAP Baking Mix calls for aluminum-free baking powder, while other recipes in this book calling for smaller amounts of baking powder do not specify; you can use either kind of baking powder in them. We have tested our recipes using Rumford or Red Star brand aluminum-free baking powder.

Chewy Chocolate Chip Cookies

Most wheat-free chocolate chip cookies are cake-like or crumbly. These cookies have a texture just like the traditional wheat-based cookies. Karo Corn Syrup is not high-fructose corn syrup and keeps the cookies chewy and moist. Do not skip chilling the dough to prevent the cookies from spreading.

2 cups uncooked old-fashioned oats
1 ⅓ cups Low-FODMAP All-Purpose Flour (page 57)
1 teaspoon baking powder
¼ teaspoon baking soda
½ scant teaspoon salt
5 tablespoons butter, melted
¾ cup plus 2 tablespoons packed light brown sugar
¼ cup Karo Light Corn Syrup (not Karo Lite)
¼ cup canola oil
1 large egg
1 large egg yolk
1 ½ teaspoons vanilla
1 ½ cups semi-sweet chocolate chips

- Grind the oats into coarse flour in a blender, food processor, or coffee mill. Stir in the Low-FODMAP All-Purpose Flour, baking powder, baking soda, and salt and set aside.
- In a large mixing bowl, with a hand mixer, beat the melted butter and brown sugar until creamy, about 1 minute. Beat in corn syrup and canola oil until smooth. Add whole egg, egg yolk, and vanilla and mix until creamy. Add flour mixture to wet ingredients and mix for 2 minutes. Fold in chocolate chips. Dough will be soft and wet. Chill until dough is firm and can be formed without sticking to hands, 45-60 minutes.
- Preheat oven to 350° F. Place oven rack slightly above the middle position. Coat a baking sheet with baking spray or oil.
- Roll dough into 1-inch balls and place 2 inches apart on baking sheet. Bake until light golden brown, 10-12 minutes. Cool 1-2 minutes, and remove cookies while still warm.

Servings: 18, 2 cookies each

Tips: If cookies cool too long on the tray, they will be hard to remove. If this happens, turn off oven, place baking sheet in warm oven for 2 minutes to soften cookies, then remove immediately. For a warm, just-baked taste, microwave cookies for 10-15 seconds before serving.

Substitutions: Substitute 1 ½ cups plus 2 tablespoons commercial oat flour for the home-ground oats.

Variations: For chewy toffee bit cookies, use English toffee bits instead of chocolate chips.

Nutrition (per serving): 182 calories, 25.3g carbohydrates, 2.5g protein, 9.1g total fat, 70mg sodium, 1.8g fiber, 44.4mg calcium.

Cranberry Scones with Orange Glaze

These scones are tasty plain or with jam or nut butter, and make an easy, portable snack. The use of yogurt that is thickened by draining (page 140) keeps these scones moist for days.

Scones:
2 ¼ cups Low-FODMAP Baking Mix (page 56)
¼ teaspoon baking soda
2 tablespoons whole chia seeds
½ cup granulated sugar
Zest of 1 orange
5 tablespoons cold, unsalted butter, cut into ½-inch pieces
1 large egg
¾ cup plain, thickened lactose-free yogurt (page 140)
¼ cup freshly squeezed orange juice
1 teaspoon vanilla
1 cup fresh cranberries, coarsely chopped

Tips: Fresh cranberries freeze very well in the bag. When in season, freeze several bags to have on hand year-round. Thaw before chopping by placing measured amount in a bowl of warm water.

Time saver: Sprinkle scones with raw sugar crystals before baking and omit glaze.

Orange Glaze:
1 cup confectioners' sugar
1-2 tablespoons orange juice
½ teaspoon orange zest
¼ teaspoon vanilla

- Preheat oven to 400° F. Place oven rack one position above middle if possible. Lightly coat a baking sheet with baking spray or oil.
- Combine baking mix, baking soda, chia seeds, sugar, and zest in a food processor or large mixing bowl. Add butter and pulse several times (or cut in by hand) until flour mixture resembles coarse breadcrumbs.
- Beat egg in a small bowl. Stir in yogurt, orange juice, and vanilla until combined. Add wet mixture to dry ingredients and stir or pulse very lightly 2-3 times, just until a very thick dough that holds its shape forms. Fold in the chopped cranberries by hand.
- Spoon about ⅓ cup of dough onto baking sheet to form 10 scones; leave the tops a bit craggy and uneven. Bake until light golden brown, 13-15 minutes. Remove from oven, cool 5 minutes, and transfer scones to a cooling rack.
- While scones are baking, combine glaze ingredients in a small bowl, using only 1 tablespoon of orange juice, and mix until smooth. Add more orange juice a teaspoon at a time until the glaze is pourable. Turn cooled scones upside down, dip the top into the glaze and let the excess drip off. Turn scones right size up and allow glaze to dry before storing.

Nutrition (per serving): 231 calories, 38.4g carbohydrates, 3.8g protein, 7.4g total fat, 326.3mg sodium, 2.6g fiber, 132.5mg calcium.

Kabocha Squash Pie with Gingersnap Crust

Kabocha squash is especially low in FODMAPs and tastes great in pie. Be sure to allow extra time to prepare the squash puree (see tips) and par-bake the crust.

1 ¾ cups cooked kabocha squash (2 pounds squash)
¾ cup packed light brown sugar
1 tablespoon plus 1 teaspoon cornstarch
2 teaspoons pumpkin pie spice (or make your own, see substitutions, page 76)
1 ½ teaspoons vanilla
⅛ teaspoon salt
2 large eggs
1 large egg yolk
1 cup lactose-free whole milk
1 recipe Easy Cookie Crumb Crust, par-baked (next page)

- Preheat oven to 350° F.
- Puree kabocha squash in a food processor until very smooth or beat squash with an electric hand mixer in a large bowl. Add brown sugar, cornstarch, spice, vanilla, and salt and beat until smooth. Add eggs and yolk and mix until smooth. Stir in milk.
- Pour filling into crumb crust to the top edge of the crust. There will be extra filling. Pour extra into oiled ramekins until ¾ full. Bake pie until the center is set, 45-50 minutes. Ramekins will be done in 20-25 minutes. Chill pie before serving.

Servings: 10

Tips: Pierce kabocha in 2 places with a sharp knife. Place on a microwave safe plate and cook on high power until a knife inserts easily through to the middle, 6-10 minutes. Cut horizontally in half. Remove seeds and strings and scoop out flesh. Mash with a fork or potato masher. Puree can be frozen.

Variations: Skip the crust and bake the filling in a 1-quart casserole for a flan-like dessert.

Nutrition, including crust (per serving): 256 calories, 44.8g carbohydrate, 3.7g fat, 3.7g protein, 145.5mg sodium, 1.9g fiber, 82.2mg calcium.

Easy Cookie Crumb Crust

This crust requires little effort and can be made with any type of crispy, low-FODMAP cookies.

6 ounces low-FODMAP gingersnaps
2 tablespoons granulated sugar
¼ cup melted butter (½ stick)

- Preheat oven to 350° F. Lightly coat a 9-inch pie pan with baking spray or oil. Pulse cookies, sugar, and melted butter in a food processor until ground to a crumb-like texture (about 1 ½ cups). Alternatively, crush cookies in a zip-top bag (leave a tiny opening) with a rolling pin or a saucepan and combine remaining ingredients. Press crumbs over the bottom and up the sides of the pie pan. To par-bake, place in the preheated oven for about 5 minutes, just until set; do not brown.

Servings: 10

Tips: If using soft cookies, dry the cookies in a 300° F oven. Crumble cookies until pea-sized and bake, stirring periodically until dry, 15-25 minutes. Time depends on cookie moisture. Cool and process into crumbs. When using crust for a pie with a no-bake filling, bake crust fully until golden brown, 6-9 minutes total, and cool before filling.

Substitutions: Other low-FODMAP cookies, animal crackers, or shortbread can be substituted for the gingersnaps.

Nutrition (per serving): 121 calories, 15.6g carbohydrates, 1g protein, 6.3g total fat, 144mg sodium, <1g fiber, 14.5mg calcium.

Peanut Butter Chocolate Chip Bars

If you have made the Low-FODMAP Baking Mix, you are 10 minutes away from baking these tasty, rich bars. Parchment paper makes it much easier to get these bars out of the pan, so be sure to keep some on hand.

1 cup Low-FODMAP Baking Mix (page 56)
4 tablespoons butter (½ stick)
⅔ cup creamy peanut butter
1 cup packed light brown sugar
1 large egg
2 teaspoons vanilla
½ cup semi-sweet chocolate chips

- Preheat oven to 350° F. Coat a 9 x 9-inch baking pan with baking spray or oil. Cut a piece of parchment paper 9 x 15-inches; place parchment in pan and press to adhere.
- Measure peanut butter and butter into a large microwave safe bowl. Cook on high power just until butter and peanut butter are melted, about 1 minute. Do not overheat. Stir until smooth. Stir in brown sugar, vanilla, and salt to form a grainy batter. If mixture is very hot, allow it to cool a few minutes. Stir in egg until completely incorporated. Add flour and stir until a very thick, dough-like batter forms. Stir in chips.
- Scrape batter into prepared pan. Pat dough into pan, spreading it evenly with hands to edges and corners. Bake until golden brown along edges and a toothpick inserted in the center comes out clean, 20-25 minutes. Cool on wire rack. Use the parchment overhang to lift bar out of pan and cut into 20 pieces.

Servings: 20

Substitutions: If using unsalted butter, add ¼ teaspoon salt to the dough.

Nutrition (per serving): 162 calories, 20.5g carbohydrates, 3.1g protein, 8.3g total fat, 136.5mg sodium, 1.1g fiber, 35.5mg calcium.

Pecan Pie Meringues

One day Lisa decided to try brown sugar instead of white sugar in a meringue recipe. We think you will agree that the switch takes the confections to another level. Meringues do take a long time to bake, but the prep is fast and easy.

> 4 large egg whites, room temperature
> 1 cup packed light brown sugar
> ¼ teaspoon cream of tartar
> ¼ teaspoon salt
> 1 ½ teaspoons vanilla
> 1 cup coarsely chopped toasted pecans

- Preheat oven to 200° F.
- Line two baking sheets with parchment paper or foil. Separate cold eggs into glass, ceramic, or stainless bowls. Do not let any yolk get into the whites, and do not use a plastic bowl as small nicks can hide bits of oil that will prevent the whites from whipping.
- Warm egg whites by placing the bowl of whites into a larger bowl filled with warm water until they come to room temperature.
- Remove bowl of whites from water bath and beat on medium until foamy. Add cream of tartar and salt. Beat until soft peaks form and flop over when beaters are lifted. Add brown sugar 2 tablespoons at a time while beating, until each addition is well mixed. The whites will turn thick and shiny. Add vanilla and continue beating until a bit of meringue rubbed between the fingers is no longer gritty, 2-3 minutes. A few sugar particles are fine. Gently fold in pecans.
- Use two spoons, one to scoop up 2 tablespoons of meringue, and the other to scrape off the meringue onto parchment 1 ½ inches apart. Smooth down any large peaks. Bake for 2 hours. Turn off heat, open oven door and let meringues cool to room temperature. Store in an airtight container.

Servings: 20 servings, 2 meringues each

Tips: Eggs separate best when cold but whip up best when warm.

Substitutions: If you don't have cream of tartar on hand, use ¼ teaspoon lemon juice or white vinegar instead.

Variations: For chocolate chip or toffee meringues, fold in ⅓ cup mini chocolate chips, coarsely chopped dark chocolate, or toffee chips in addition to the pecans. For chocolate-pecan meringues, fold in 3 tablespoons of cocoa powder along with the pecans. For maple flavor, add ½ teaspoon maple extract in addition to vanilla.

Nutrition (per serving): 84 calories, 11.7g carbohydrates, 1.2g protein, 3.9g total fat, 43.3mg sodium, <1g fiber, 13.5mg calcium.

Double-Concentrated Simple Syrup

Simple syrup is really simple to make. Double-concentrated simple syrup adds sweetness without diluting other flavors.

> ½ cup sugar
> ¼ cup water

- Stir sugar and water together in a small saucepan over medium heat until sugar is dissolved, about 3 minutes. Cool before using. Keeps in the refrigerator in a glass jar for several months. Reheat if sugar crystals form.
- Use simple syrup in iced tea or coffee, smoothies, or in mixed drinks, where it instantly dissolves in cold liquids.

Yield: ½ cup

Nutrition (entire recipe): 387 calories, 100g carbohydrates, 0g protein, 0g total fat, 0mg sodium, 0g fiber, 1mg calcium.

Pina Colada Granita

This incredibly simple non-dairy dessert is refreshing and elegant. Plan ahead as it takes several hours to freeze. For a rich taste, use full-fat canned coconut milk (not coconut water, cream or "beverage").

3 cups unsweetened 100% pineapple juice
1 (14-ounce) can coconut milk
1 teaspoon vanilla
1 tablespoon lime juice
1 teaspoon vanilla extract
⅓ cup Double-Concentrated Simple Syrup
   (preceding page)
Toasted coconut flakes (optional)

- Stir all ingredients (except toasted coconut) together in a large bowl until well blended. Pour into a shallow 1 ½-quart glass or ceramic dish. Do not use metal. Place in the freezer.
- After 2-3 hours, use a fork to scrape ice crystals from the edges toward the center, to create shards of granita. Break up any large chunks that have formed. Repeat this process every hour until granita is completely frozen and flaked, 3-4 hours total. Serve immediately in wine or martini glasses topped with a toasted coconut flakes.

Servings: 12

Tips: Store granita covered in an airtight container for several weeks. Re-flake granita before serving.

Substitutions: Light coconut milk can be used in place of full-fat coconut milk, but add a ½ teaspoon coconut extract, as the coconut flavor of light coconut milk is less pronounced.

Nutrition (per serving): 116 calories, 13.8g carbohydrates, <1g protein, 7g total fat, 5.5mg sodium, <1g fiber, 9.9mg calcium.

Creamy Lemon No-Bake Cheesecake

This tart filling is not baked. Neufchatel cheese does contain lactose; however, small servings are tolerated by most people with IBS. Allow time to fully bake and cool the crust before continuing with the recipe.

1 recipe Sugar Cookie Tart Crust (page 70)
12-ounce block Neufchatel cream cheese
⅓ cup confectioners' sugar
1 teaspoon vanilla
¾ cup lemon curd (found in jars near jams and
   jellies)
1 pound strawberries, hulled and halved
   lengthwise
1 cup blueberries
½ cup strawberry or raspberry jelly (optional for
   glaze)

- Preheat the oven to 350° F.
- Bake crust completely until lightly golden, about 25-28 minutes. Cool crust to room temperature before filling.
- Beat Neufchatel cheese until soft. Beat in confectioners' sugar and vanilla until smooth. Fold in lemon curd until mixed. Spread filling evenly over cooled tart crust. Arrange strawberries cut side down in concentric circles starting at the outer edge and working inward. Leave a 5-inch circle in the middle of the tart and fill with blueberries. Garnish with a whole strawberry in the center.

Servings: 12

Tips: Brushing a glaze on the berries adds a nice shine but is not necessary. Melt ½ cup strawberry or raspberry jelly in a saucepan or microwave until liquid. Use a pastry brush to lightly coat berries with melted jam. This tart also works well with raspberries or a combination of all three berries.

Nutrition facts for crust plus filling (per serving): 379 calories, 48.7g carbohydrates, 6g protein, 18.9g total fat, 191.5mg sodium, 2.2g fiber, 44.5mg calcium.

Why do some of our recipes call for xanthan gum?

Xanthan gum works wonders in Low-FODMAP baking. It provides binding, structure and stretchiness that are lacking without the gluten from wheat. A serving of most baked goods in this book contains about 1/12th – 1/24th of a teaspoon of xanthan gum. It is not a FODMAP, yet some people report they don't tolerate it well. If you prefer not to use it, substitute 2 teaspoons of ground chia seeds in the Low-FODMAP Baking Mix (page 56). However, be aware that all of the recipes in this book were tested with xanthan gum, so your results may vary.

Lemon Olive Oil Cake

This moist lemony cake uses heart-healthy olive oil in place of butter.

Cake:
½ cup whole toasted almonds (2 ounces)
1 cup sugar, divided
1 cup Low-FODMAP All-Purpose Flour (page 57)
1 ½ teaspoons baking powder
¼ teaspoon salt
½ teaspoon xanthan gum
1 tablespoon lemon zest
2 large eggs
⅓ cup extra virgin olive oil
½ cup lactose-free yogurt
1 teaspoon almond extract
¼ cup fresh lemon juice
Lemon Glaze:
½ cup confectioners' sugar
1 tablespoon plus 2 teaspoons lemon juice

Tips: If you don't have parchment paper, spray and flour pan sides and bottom, tapping out excess flour.

Variations: Skip the glaze and dust with confectioners' sugar instead. Serve with berry mix (sliced strawberries, blueberries, and raspberries).

Nutrition (per serving): 266 calories, 36.5g carbohydrates, 4.4g protein, 12.3g total fat, 160.1mg sodium, 2g fiber, 102mg calcium.

- Preheat oven to 350° F. Coat a 9-inch cake pan with baking spray or oil. Line the bottom of the pan with a circle of parchment paper and spray the paper.
- Pulse toasted almonds and ½ cup sugar together in a food processor in short 5-10 second bursts to grind nuts until they resemble coarse flour. Add flour, baking powder, salt, xanthan gum, and zest and pulse to combine.
- In a mixing bowl, beat eggs with an electric mixer. Beat in remaining ½ cup sugar until mixture is lemon colored, about 2 minutes. With beater on low, drizzle in olive oil until incorporated, then mix in yogurt and almond extract. Slowly drizzle in lemon juice. Add flour and almond mixture and beat for one minute on medium speed.
- Pour batter into cake pan and bake in the middle of the oven until light golden brown and a toothpick inserted in the center comes out clean, 30-40 minutes. Cool cake in pan. Turn cake out onto serving platter and peel off parchment.
- Stir glaze ingredients together in a small bowl to make a thin, pourable glaze. Drizzle glaze over cake, letting it run over the sides. Serve with berries.

Servings: 10

Russian Tea Cakes

These cookies, also known as Mexican Wedding Cakes, are one of the first recipes Lisa adapted to a wheat-free version over 20 years ago. They are not only easy to make, but the dough is very forgiving and allows for substitution of any low-FODMAP nuts and flavorings. Kids love to help shape the cookies and roll them in powdered sugar. Take the time to toast the nuts, as the flavor of the cookie goes from good to great. The recipe is easily halved or doubled. Sweet rice flour, also known as glutinous rice flour, can be found in Asian markets.

1 cup toasted almonds
1 ¼ cups Low-FODMAP All-Purpose Flour (page 57)
½ cup sweet rice flour
¼ teaspoon salt
1 teaspoon xanthan gum
1 cup unsalted butter, room temperature (2 sticks)
⅔ cup confectioners' sugar
1 egg yolk
1 teaspoon vanilla extract
1 teaspoon almond extract
1-1 ½ cups additional confectioners' sugar for coating cookies

- Preheat oven to 350° F.
- Pulse toasted nuts in a food processor until they are the texture of very coarse bread crumbs, or chop by hand. Combine nuts and flours, salt, and xanthan gum and set aside.
- Beat butter and ⅔ cup confectioners' sugar together with an electric mixer until creamy. Beat in egg yolk and extracts. Add flour and nut mixture and beat until combined, scraping sides occasionally. The dough will have the texture of soft children's play clay. Cover and refrigerate dough for 45-60 minutes, or up to 24 hours.
- Form dough into 1-inch balls and place 2 inches apart on an ungreased baking sheet. Bake just until the bottoms of the cookies are a golden brown (lift and peek), 12-14 minutes. Cool on the baking sheet for 2-3 minutes, then remove to a wire rack to cool. While cookies are still slightly warm, place 1 cup confectioners' sugar in a small bowl and roll each cookie in sugar to coat well. Cool to room temperature on wire rack and roll again in the confectioners' sugar, adding more if needed. Cookies can be frozen for several months in an airtight container.

Servings: 15, 2 cookies each

Tips: To toast nuts, preheat oven to 350° F. Toast nuts on a baking sheet until light golden brown, about 10-15 minutes, stirring midway.

Substitutions: ½ cup additional Low-FODMAP All-Purpose Flour can be used in place of ½ cup sweet rice flour.

Variations: Toasted pecans, walnuts, or hazelnuts can be used in place of almonds; omit almond extract. For spice cookies, add ½ teaspoon cinnamon, ¼ teaspoon nutmeg, and ⅛ teaspoon cloves. For lemon cookies, add 2-3 teaspoons finely grated lemon zest and ½ teaspoon lemon extract. For chocolate dipped batons, shape dough into logs, about 2 x ½-inch. Bake as directed and let cookies cool to room temperature. Melt 1 cup semi-sweet chocolate morsels in a microwave-safe bowl on high power in 30-second increments, stirring each time. Dip half of each cookie in chocolate and place on parchment-lined baking sheet until chocolate sets (chilling speeds it up). For a pretty presentation, dip the other half of the cookie in powdered sugar. Cookies can be stored once the chocolate has set.

Nutrition (per serving): 207 calories, 11.4g carbohydrates, 2.9g protein, 17.4g total fat, 48.2mg sodium, 1.8g fiber, 30.3mg calcium.

Strawberry Rhubarb Cobbler

This dessert reminds us of summer, even though it can be made year-round, if you plan ahead and stock your freezer with frozen rhubarb and berries.

Filling:
1 cup sugar
2 tablespoons cornstarch
5 cups sliced strawberries (1 ¼ pounds)
5 cups sliced rhubarb (1 ¼ pounds)
Zest from one lemon
Topping:
2 cups Low-FODMAP Baking Mix (page 56)
¾ cup plus 1 tablespoon granulated sugar, divided
½ cup cold butter (1 stick), cut into small pieces
1 large egg
⅓ cup lactose-free milk
1 teaspoon almond extract

- Preheat oven to 375° F. Coat a 9 x 13 x 2-inch baking pan with baking spray or oil.
- In a large bowl, combine sugar and cornstarch. Add sliced strawberries, rhubarb, and zest and mix well.
- Pour into prepared pan and bake until fruit has softened and juices have thickened, about 25 minutes. Remove pan from oven.
- While fruit is baking, prepare topping. Combine baking mix and ¾ cup sugar. Cut butter into dry ingredients using a pastry blender until mixture is crumbly. Lightly beat egg, milk, and extract together in a small bowl and pour over flour mixture. Mix lightly, just until a wet batter forms.
- Drop batter by golf-ball-sized spoonfuls evenly over partially cooked fruit. Batter will melt together during baking. Sprinkle topping with 1 tablespoon sugar and bake one rack below middle position (bottom third), until topping is firm and golden brown, 25-30 minutes.

Servings: 12

Tips: If you don't have a pastry blender, use two table knives to cut butter into the flour until crumbly. Buy rhubarb in season, cut it into ¼-inch pieces and freeze.

Substitutions: Add ⅛ teaspoon of salt if using unsalted butter.

Variations: Reduce sugar to ¾ cup if you prefer a tart filling. For berry cobbler, replace rhubarb with more berries. Reduce sugar in filling to ⅔-¾ cup, depending on preferred sweetness.

Nutrition (per serving): 295 calories, 52g carbohydrates, 3.5g protein, 9.2g total fat, 242.5mg sodium, 3.5g fiber, 142.3mg calcium.

Wheat-free baking and high protein ingredients

High-protein ingredients vastly improve the texture of baked goods made with alternative flours. Add protein in the form of nut flours, nut butters, eggs, lactose-free cow's milk, plain yogurt, cheese, or cottage cheese. During the elimination phase of the low-FODMAP diet, stick with lactose-free options. Later, as you begin to test your tolerance, you may find you can tolerate small amounts of lactose-containing products used in baking. An entire recipe calling for ½ cup of yogurt may contain less than a gram of lactose per serving. Most people with IBS can tolerate that amount. Note that non-dairy milks are not good protein sources.

Chocolate Decadence Tart

This is a make-ahead recipe. In addition to allowing time for the crust to be par-baked and cooled, the filled tart needs to be chilled before serving.

1 recipe Sugar Cookie Tart Crust (below)
1 cup heavy cream
1 teaspoon vanilla extract
1 ½ cups semi-sweet chocolate morsels
¼ teaspoon salt
2 eggs
Whipped cream or raspberries (optional)

Nutrition facts for crust plus filling (per serving): 366 calories, 38.3g carbohydrates, 4.1g protein, 23.6g total fat, 146.2mg sodium, 2.2g fiber, 32.8mg calcium.

- Preheat the oven to 350° F.
- Par-bake the crust until it is firm, but still pale in color, 18-20 minutes. Remove from the oven and set aside.
- Reduce oven temperature to 325° F.
- Stir cream and vanilla together in a small saucepan over medium-low heat until cream bubbles around the edges. Remove saucepan from heat, add chocolate, and let sit for one minute. Stir until chocolate is melted, then stir in salt.
- Beat eggs in a medium bowl. Whisk one third of the chocolate cream mixture into the eggs until smooth. Scrape the egg-chocolate mixture back into saucepan, and stir until smooth.
- Pour chocolate filling into the par-baked crust and bake until the filling is set and the center wiggles slightly when the tart is moved, 20-25 minutes. Remove from oven to a rack and cool. Refrigerate tart until cold and firm. Remove tart ring, cut into wedges and serve with whipped cream or fresh raspberries if desired.

Servings: 12

Sugar Cookie Tart Crust

This sweet, low-FODMAP crust tastes like sugar cookies. It doesn't need to be rolled out so it is easy to make.

1 large egg
1 teaspoon almond extract
1 teaspoon vanilla extract
1 ½ cups Low-FODMAP All-Purpose Flour (page 57)
½ cup sugar
¼ teaspoon salt
½ teaspoon xanthan gum
½ cup unsalted butter (1 stick), cut into 8 pieces

Nutrition (per serving): 170 calories, 22.5g carbohydrates, 1.7g protein, 8.4g total fat, 61.8mg sodium, <1g fiber, 7.9mg calcium

Variations: Replace ½–¾ cup of flour with an equal amount of ground nuts (almonds, pecans, or walnuts)

- Coat a 10-inch tart pan (with removable bottom) with baking spray or oil. Beat egg and extracts together in a bowl and set aside.
- Pulse flour, sugar, salt, and xanthan gum in a food processor. Add butter and pulse until mixture looks like fine breadcrumbs. With processor running, pour egg into crust and pulse until a thick dough forms. Place spoonfuls of dough evenly around the bottom of tart pan. Cover dough with a piece of plastic wrap and press dough evenly over the bottom and up the sides of the tart pan. Freeze crust for 30 minutes. See recipe above for baking instructions.

Servings: 12

Pizza Crust and Focaccia

Lisa has tried many wheat-free pizza crusts, and most were crunchy, dry, or crumbly. After many trials, she finally found the "real" pizza crust she was looking for. The recipe makes 2 par-baked crusts—use one now and freeze the other. Even though the recipe is easy, there are several steps followed by rest periods, so plan ahead, and be sure to have parchment paper on hand. It will be worth the effort.

> 3 cups Low-FODMAP Baking Mix (page 56)
> 1 tablespoon plus 1 teaspoon whole chia seeds (or
>   2 tablespoons ground chia seeds)
> ¼ teaspoon salt
> ¾ cup lactose-free milk
> ½ cup plus 2 tablespoons water
> 1 tablespoon active dry yeast
> 4 tablespoons plus two teaspoons extra-virgin
>   olive oil for baking

- Prepare 2 large baking sheets or 10" or larger pizza pans by lightly coating each pan with baking spray or oil.
- Combine Low-FODMAP Baking Mix, chia seed, and salt in the mixing bowl of a stand mixer and stir to combine.
- In a medium microwave safe bowl, combine milk and water. Heat in the microwave until lukewarm, but not more than 115° F. Sprinkle yeast over warm milk, stir, and let sit for 3 minutes. Remove ½ cup of the Low-FODMAP Baking Mix from the mixing bowl and add it to the warm milk and yeast mixture to make a sponge. Stir to combine (some lumps are fine) and let it sit for 30 minutes. The sponge should smell yeast-like, bubble up, and nearly double in volume. Pour sponge into the mixing bowl and add 2 tablespoons olive oil. Beat on medium speed for 4 minutes. Let the dough rest for 20 minutes. It will be a very thick batter.
- Turn oven to lowest setting, usually 150-170° F. When at temperature, *turn oven off*.
- Cut two pieces of parchment paper large enough to completely cover both baking pans. Trace a 10" circle (most dinner plates are about 10") with a pencil on each piece of parchment. Turn paper over and place on baking sheet, pressing to adhere. Pour 1 tablespoon plus 1 teaspoon of olive oil inside each parchment circle and spread oil with fingers throughout the circle to the edge. Scrape half of the dough into the center of each circle. Lightly coat hands with some of the olive oil on the parchment and pat dough evenly to the edges of the circle, smoothing edges.
- Place pans in the warm oven (make sure oven is off) until dough is puffy, 15-20 minutes. Remove dough from oven and turn oven to 400° F. Gently pinch the edges of the crust to form a lip. When oven is at temperature, par-bake crusts in the middle of the oven until the top of the crust is firm but pale and the bottom is a medium golden brown, about 8 minutes. If both pans won't fit on the middle rack of the oven, par-bake one crust at a time.

Servings: 16, ⅛ of a 10" pizza crust each

Tips: Place toppings on pizza and bake for an additional 10-12 minutes until crust is golden brown around the edges and cheese is melted. If the crust is getting too dark and toppings aren't cooked, turn oven to broil. Move pizza to the top oven rack and broil until cheese is melted.

Variations: For focaccia bread, add ⅓ cup very thinly sliced scallion greens, and 1 tablespoon finely chopped fresh rosemary (or 1 ½ teaspoons dried, crushed rosemary leaves) into the dry ingredients. Follow recipe above through the rise in the warm oven. Do not par-bake. Make several indentations lightly with your fingers. Drizzle crusts with 1-2 tablespoons garlic-infused oil and sprinkle with coarse salt, pepper, and additional rosemary. Add sliced Kalamata olives if desired and bake at 400° F until golden brown all over, 18-20 minutes. Serve warm. Focaccia can be reheated in the microwave or in the oven.

Time savers: Freeze the second crust after par-baking and cooling (do not add toppings). Double wrap tightly before freezing. To finish, preheat oven to 400° F. Remove crust from the freezer, add toppings and bake as above.

Nutrition (per ⅛ of 10" pizza crust): 136 calories, 20.8g carbohydrates, 2.5g protein, 5.1g total fat, 269mg sodium, 1.6g fiber, 88.6mg calcium.

> **Cornmeal and low-FODMAP baking**
>
> Cornmeal adds a distinctive corn taste, yellow color, and heavy texture to baked goods. It can also add crunch if coarse or stone-ground cornmeal is used. Quaker cornmeal is medium-fine. Extra-fine cornmeal (GOYA brand) is more flour-like and can be found in Hispanic sections of supermarkets. The first time you make a recipe calling for cornmeal, use the type of grind called for—results vary quite a bit with substitutions.

Corn Bread

This recipe is very forgiving and goes well with a variety of soups and stews.

1 ½ cups stone-ground cornmeal
1 cup Low-FODMAP All-Purpose Flour (page 57)
½ cup granulated sugar
1 ½ teaspoons baking powder
½ teaspoon baking soda
¾ teaspoon salt
½ teaspoon xanthan gum
1 ½ cups lactose-free milk
1 tablespoon white vinegar
2 large eggs
¼ cup butter, melted

- Preheat oven to 425° F. Coat a 9 x 9 x 2-inch pan with baking spray or oil.
- Stir cornmeal, flour, sugar, baking powder, baking soda, salt, and xanthan gum together in a medium bowl and set aside.
- Combine milk and vinegar in a small bowl and let sit for 5 minutes. Whisk eggs and melted butter into milk. Add the wet ingredients to the dry mixture and stir until no lumps remain.
- Pour batter into pan and bake until cornbread is light golden brown, 18-20 minutes.

Servings: 16

Substitutions: Oil can be used in place of butter.

Variations: For cake-like cornbread, use a medium-fine grind of cornmeal (ex: Quaker brand) in place of the stone-ground, and add more liquid. For a crunchier, full cornmeal flavor, increase the amount of stone-ground cornmeal and decrease the flour by the same amount, but decrease the liquid. For cheese cornbread, add 1 cup shredded sharp cheddar. For muffins, preheat oven to 400 F. Fill greased muffin cups ¾ full and bake 12-15 minutes.

Timesavers: Make several corn bread mixes in zip-top bags and you can have cornbread in the oven in 5 minutes. Stand several open bags upright in a bowl. Place 1 ½ cups of cornmeal, 1 cup Low-FODMAP All-Purpose Flour, and so on, in each bag assembly-line style, adding all dry ingredients in recipe. On the label, list the wet ingredient amounts to be added later, baking temperature, and time. Store in a cool, dry place, preferably in a refrigerator or freezer.

Nutrition (per serving): 133 calories, 21.4g carbohydrates, 3.1g protein, 4.3g total fat, 221.4mg sodium, 1.3g fiber, 59.6mg calcium

Sweet Potato Biscuits

These biscuits were adapted from a *Bon Appétit* recipe; they make a great Thanksgiving or winter dinner accompaniment or a tasty snack. This recipe was tested with Quaker cornmeal.

½ cup lactose-free milk
1 ½ teaspoons white vinegar or lemon juice
1 ½ cups Low-FODMAP Baking Mix (page 56),
    plus extra for forming biscuits
½ cup yellow medium-grind cornmeal
½ teaspoon baking soda
2 tablespoons packed light brown sugar
6 tablespoons cold unsalted butter, cut into 12
    pieces
1 cup cooked, mashed sweet potato
½ cup coarsely chopped, toasted pecan halves

Tips: For cooked, mashed sweet potato, pierce a large, unpeeled sweet potato with a fork and microwave on high power until soft, 4-7 minutes. Cut and scoop out flesh and mash with a fork until smooth.

Nutrition (per serving): 138 calories, 17.1g carbohydrates, 1.9g protein, 7.4g total fat, 163.2mg sodium, 1.5g fiber, 53mg calcium.

- Preheat oven to 400° F. and move oven rack to one position above middle. Coat a baking sheet with baking spray or oil.
- Mix milk and vinegar in a small bowl and set aside.
- Measure baking mix, cornmeal, baking soda, and brown sugar into the bowl of a food processor and pulse to combine. Add butter and pulse until flour resembles coarse meal. Add sweet potato and milk mixture and pulse quickly to blend. Dough will be very wet. Add pecans and pulse quickly 2-3 times.
- Generously coat a surface with 1-2 tablespoons of Baking Mix. Scrape dough onto the floured surface and sprinkle top of the dough with just enough flour to keep hands from sticking, 1-2 teaspoons. Gently knead dough 3-4 times until smooth, adding small amounts of flour if needed. Pat dough into an 8-inch square. Dust a large knife with flour and cut into 16 squares. Transfer biscuits to the baking tray and bake until biscuits are golden brown on the bottom and a toothpick inserted into center comes out clean, 15-20 minutes. Serve warm, with butter. Biscuits can be reheated in a microwave on high power for about 15 seconds. Biscuits freeze well.

Servings: 16

Two ways to toast nuts
Toasting nuts really amps up the flavor and crunch.

1. Just a few nuts? Toast them in a dry skillet over medium heat, stirring constantly for 1-3 minutes. Beware, nuts burn easily.
2. Oven-toasted nuts yield better flavor and more even browning. Preheat oven to 350° F. Spread whole nuts in a single layer on a baking sheet and toast until light to medium golden brown, 10-15 minutes, stirring half-way through. Chopped or small nuts will toast faster, 7-10 minutes. Check frequently near the end as nuts can burn quickly and will continue to brown even after removing from the oven.

Tips for serving and storing low-FODMAP baked goods

Baked goods made with alternative flours taste great the day they are made, but because they lack gluten they dry out more quickly than regular baked goods. They tend to get moldy faster as well. To keep them fresh, tasty and moist, follow these simple tips:

1. After cooling, but no more than 24-hours after baking, refrigerate for up to one week, or freeze.
2. Cut larger items like Banana Bread or Corn Bread into individual servings and double wrap before freezing, excluding as much air as possible.
3. Warm refrigerated or frozen baked goods briefly before serving to restore moisture, reduce crumbling and bring back that just-baked taste and texture. Microwave a single serving for 10-30 seconds on high power or heat foil-wrapped portion in the oven until soft and warm. Don't overheat them or they will become mushy.

Breakfast

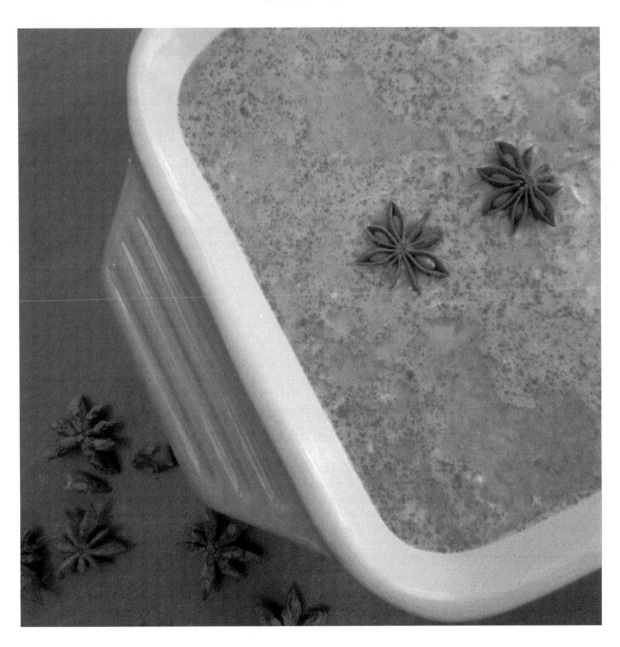

Baked "Pumpkin Pie" Oatmeal

This warm, filling breakfast uses kabocha squash, a low-FODMAP squash which tastes very similar to pumpkin. The dish can be put together the night before, refrigerated, and baked in the morning.

3 large eggs
3 cups lactose-free milk
½ cup packed light brown sugar
1 cup cooked mashed kabocha squash
2 teaspoons vanilla
2 ¼ cups old fashioned, rolled oats
2 teaspoons pumpkin pie spice
1 teaspoon baking powder
⅛ teaspoon salt
Star anise (optional)

- Preheat oven to 375° F. Coat a 2-quart baking dish with baking spray or oil.
- Beat eggs in a large bowl. Mix in milk, brown sugar, squash and vanilla. Stir in oats, pumpkin pie spice, baking powder and salt. Pour into baking pan, decorate with star anise (optional) and bake in the middle of the oven until golden brown on top and cooked through the middle, 45-60 min. Remove star anise before serving or storing in the refrigerator.

Servings: 9

Substitutions: If you don't have pumpkin pie spice on hand, substitute ½ teaspoon ground ginger, 1 teaspoon cinnamon, ¼ teaspoon each grated nutmeg and ground allspice, ⅛ teaspoon ground cloves.

Variations: For maple oatmeal, replace brown sugar with ½ cup maple syrup added to wet ingredients. Add ½ teaspoon maple extract. Reduce milk to 2 ¾ cups. For banana oatmeal, omit kabocha squash and add 1 cup mashed bananas (2-3 bananas). Reduce brown sugar to ⅓ cup.

Time Savers: For a quick weekday breakfast, bake in advance and reheat, covered in the oven, or cut into individual pieces and microwave.

Nutrition (per serving): 274 calories, 44.1g carbohydrates, 11.6g protein, 6g total fat, 148.3mg sodium, 4.5g fiber, 175.4mg calcium.

Tips for preparing kabocha squash

Kabocha squash is low-FODMAP and readily available, often mixed in with the buttercup squash at the grocery store, but minus the "turban" shape on the bottom of the squash. Pierce kabocha in 2 places with a sharp knife. Place on a microwave-safe plate and cook on high power. For a puree, cook until a knife inserts easily through to the middle, 6-10 minutes. Cut horizontally in half. Remove seeds and strings and scoop out flesh. Mash with a fork or potato masher. Extra squash can be frozen. Kabocha skin is tender and edible when fully cooked, so if you will be using the squash in a soup or stew, microwave only long enough to allow the squash to be easily chopped, then remove seeds and toss pieces in the pot, skin and all.

Lemon "Poppy" Pancakes

These lemony, lightly sweetened pancakes use chia seeds, which look similar to poppy seeds, to improve the texture and add fiber. Serve with strawberries, blueberries, yogurt, jam, a dusting of confectioners' sugar, or Wild Blueberry Syrup (page 131).

1 cup Low-FODMAP Baking Mix (page 56)
3 tablespoons granulated sugar
1 tablespoon lemon zest
2 large eggs
¾ cup lactose-free milk
¾ cup lactose-free cottage cheese
2 tablespoons whole chia seeds
3 tablespoons fresh lemon juice
1 teaspoon vanilla

- Combine Low-FODMAP Baking Mix, sugar, and lemon zest in a medium-sized mixing bowl and set aside. Beat eggs lightly in a separate bowl. Mix in milk, cottage cheese, chia seeds, lemon juice, and vanilla. Add wet ingredients to flour mixture and stir until no streaks of flour remain. The mixture will be lumpy from the cottage cheese. Let batter sit for 5 minutes. Batter will be slightly thicker than regular pancake batter, but pourable. Add additional milk if necessary.
- Heat skillet on medium-low heat; these need a lower heat than regular pancakes. Coat pan with baking spray or oil. Pour batter to form a 3-inch pancake, and immediately spread batter lightly with the back of a spoon to form a 4-inch pancake. When pancake edges look dry, turn pancake over and cook on the other side. Pancakes can be refrigerated or frozen and reheated in a microwave or in the oven.

Servings: 8, 2 pancakes each

Tips: Lactaid is a widely available brand of lactose-free cottage cheese.

Substitutions: Lactose-free yogurt may be used in place of cottage cheese.

Nutrition (per serving): 144 calories, 22.2g carbohydrates, 6.7g protein, 3.3g total fat, 226.7mg sodium, 2.5g fiber, 118.4mg calcium.

Basic Pancakes

Kids love pancakes. Here is a basic version using Lisa's Low-FODMAP Baking Mix that lends itself well to the addition of blueberries.

1 egg
1 ¼ cup lactose-free milk
2 tablespoons canola oil or melted butter
1 teaspoon vanilla
¼ teaspoon cinnamon
1 cup plus 2 tablespoons Low-FODMAP Baking Mix (page 56)

- Beat egg in a medium mixing bowl. Whisk in milk, oil, vanilla, and cinnamon. Stir in Low-FODMAP Baking Mix until smooth (a few lumps are fine). Set aside for 5 minutes to allow batter to absorb liquid. Batter will be thick, but pourable. If too thick add additional milk a few tablespoons at a time. Stir batter again. Heat a lightly greased griddle on medium for 2-3 minutes.
- Pour about ¼ cup batter per pancake into the pan. When bubbles form around the edges of the pancake and edges look dry, turn over and cook until browned, about 1 minute. Serve with Wild Blueberry Syrup (page 131), real maple syrup, or lactose-free yogurt and fresh fruit.

Servings: 6, 2 pancakes each

Tips: Pancakes freeze well. Reheat covered in a microwave a few at a time in short 25-30 second increments. Cold or reheated pancakes make a great snack topped with nut butter.

Variations: For blueberry pancakes, fold 1 cup blueberries into batter. To quickly thaw frozen blueberries, cover with hot water in a bowl and drain before adding to batter.

Nutrition (per serving): 169 calories, 22.8g carbohydrates, 4.5g protein, 6.7g total fat, 263.5mg sodium, 1.4g fiber, 139mg calcium.

Seitan Breakfast Sausage

Seitan, made from vital wheat gluten, is a vegan meat substitute with a chewy, meaty texture. Vital wheat gluten is the stretchy protein portion of wheat flour which remains when the carbohydrates are washed away. Unseasoned seitan would taste bland, so commercial seitan is usually flavored with onions and garlic. It is very easy (and more economical) to make your own flavorful low-FODMAP version, and you can customize the taste by adding different spices. Vital wheat gluten looks like a pale yellow/beige flour and can be found in Whole Foods Markets, some supermarkets, or online. Plan ahead, as there are a few steps. This recipe was tested with Bob's Red Mill brand vital wheat gluten. *People with celiac disease should not eat seitan.*

Seitan:
1 ¼ cup vital wheat gluten
¼ cup oat flour
2 teaspoons mild smoked paprika
½ teaspoon ground sage
½ teaspoon ground coriander
⅛ teaspoon allspice
½ teaspoon black pepper
½ teaspoon thyme
⅛ teaspoon asafetida
3 tablespoons soy sauce
1 tablespoon 100% maple syrup
2 tablespoons Garlic- and Onion-Infused Oil
     (page 124)
¾ cup water
Simmering water:
Water to come halfway up sausages
1 tablespoon soy sauce per cup of water
1 whole leek leaf, or 3 scallions, green part only
1 bay leaf

Tips: Boiled seitan can be cut into small pieces, sautéed, and added to grains, salads, or pasta, or stir-fried. Seitan can be grilled. Try it with Barbecue Sauce (page 101). To make your own oat flour, see page 56.

Substitutions: Use 1 teaspoon liquid hickory smoke flavoring instead of 2 teaspoons of smoked paprika. Play with seasonings to make a taste you like—the combinations are endless.

Variations: Seitan can also be cut into small 1-2 inch pieces for a short simmer time (20-25 minutes). Slice roll into smaller pieces to pan fry.

Time Savers: Seitan can be frozen after simmering, so double the recipe and freeze extra.

Nutrition (per serving): 127 calories, 7.8g carbohydrates, 15.1g protein, 4.2g total fat, 231.8mg sodium, <1g fiber, 36.4mg calcium.

- Combine vital wheat gluten, oat flour, and spices in a mixing bowl and make a well in the center. Combine soy sauce, maple syrup, oil, and water in a separate small bowl. Pour wet ingredients into dry and mix with a spoon. Dough will become stiff and difficult to stir. Finish mixing dough with hands and press in remaining ingredients. The dough will be very springy, so use some force to knead it for 3 minutes. Let dough rest for 10 minutes.
- Cut dough into 8 pieces with a sharp knife. Pinch and pull dough into 4" patties or links. Sausages will puff up and lose some shape when cooked, so if you prefer to keep their shape, wrap each piece tightly in foil before boiling. Twist the foil ends of links like a Tootsie Roll. Place sausages in a saucepan and add water to come halfway up sausages. Add soy sauce, leek leaf, and bay leaf to pan. Cover loosely with the lid askew and bring to a low simmer. Do not allow the water to come to a boil. Cook at a low simmer for 35 minutes, turning pieces over midway. Add more water if needed. Sausages will expand and become firm when done. Remove sausages from broth, unwrap, and refrigerate until chilled.
- Heat 1 teaspoon of oil on medium heat, brown sausages on all sides to make a crisp exterior with a soft chewy center.

Servings: 8

Quinoa Coconut Milk Breakfast Pudding

This creamy hot breakfast is a great way to introduce quinoa to children, and it is lactose-free. It can also be eaten cold as a dessert or snack.

¾ **cup uncooked quinoa, rinsed**
1 (14-ounce) can coconut milk
½ **cup water**
3 tablespoons packed light brown sugar
1 tablespoon oat flour
¼ **teaspoon ground cinnamon**
Pinch salt
1 teaspoon vanilla
¼ **teaspoon almond or maple extract**

- Combine all ingredients in a 2-quart saucepan on medium-high heat. Bring to a boil, stirring periodically. Reduce heat to a simmer and cook, uncovered, stirring every few minutes until mixture is porridge-like and quinoa is tender, 15-20 minutes. Serve immediately.

Servings: 3

Substitutions: Any low-FODMAP flour can be used instead of oat flour to thicken this cereal and make it creamy. 3 tablespoons of maple syrup or granulated sugar can be used in place of brown sugar.

Variations: Top quinoa with 1 tablespoon toasted coconut and 2 tablespoons nuts, if desired.

Nutrition (per serving): 386 calories, 53.4g carbohydrates, 8.5g protein, 17.3g total fat, 114.6mg sodium, 8.1g fiber, 138.3mg calcium.

Main Dishes

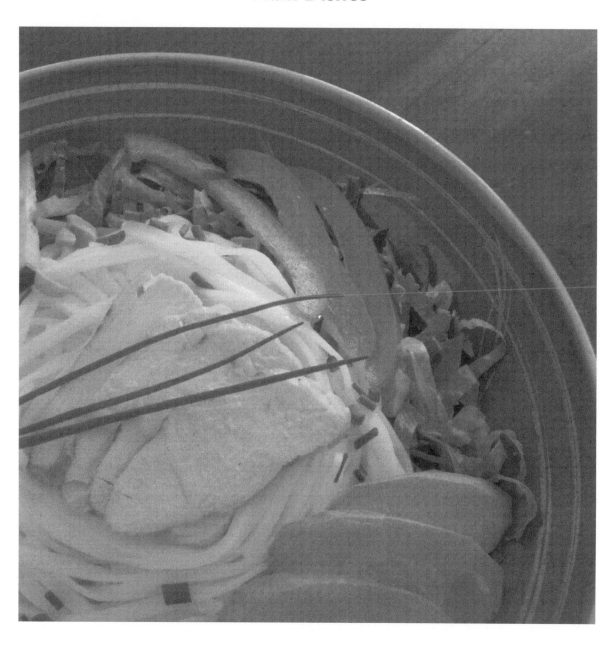

Vietnamese Rice Noodle and Chicken Salad

Vietnamese cuisine is light, tasty, and worth exploring as the dishes are often FODMAP-friendly and easy to make. Plan ahead for this recipe; you need to marinate and grill the chicken prior to assembling the salad. Do not be turned off by the pungent smell of the fish sauce – it tastes much better than it smells!

Salad Dressing and Marinade:
½ cup fish sauce
¼ cup plus 2 tablespoons packed light brown sugar
2 tablespoons garlic-infused oil
2 ½ tablespoons fresh lime juice

Grilled Chicken:
¼ teaspoon ground black pepper
1 ¼ lbs chicken breast, cut into ½-inch thick, long strips

Salad:
8 ounces thin Asian rice noodles, ¼-inch or less thick
4 cups thinly sliced lettuce
2 cups mung bean sprouts, blanched (see tips)
1 cup grated or shredded carrots
½ cucumber, peeled, thinly sliced into half moons (3 ounces)
½ bunch spearmint sprigs, washed
½ bunch cilantro sprigs, washed
4 scallions, green part only, thinly sliced
½ cup chopped roasted peanuts

- Combine fish sauce and brown sugar in a small saucepan and heat on medium, stirring just until sugar dissolves. Remove from heat and whisk in garlic-infused oil.
- For the salad dressing, measure ¼ cup of the fish sauce mixture into a small bowl. Add lime juice and 3 tablespoons of water and chill.
- Put the remaining fish sauce mixture and the black pepper in a medium bowl. Add chicken, cover, and refrigerate for at least 30 minutes. Grill or broil chicken, brushing with marinade, until cooked through and caramelized.
- Bring a large pot of water to a boil. Add rice noodles and boil 2 minutes, stirring gently to help break apart noodle bundle. Turn heat off and let sit 2 minutes, stirring once. Remove a few strands to taste. Noodles should be soft and chewy, but not mushy. Thin rice vermicelli may be done at this point. If not, leave another minute and taste again, repeating every minute until done. Medium thickness noodles will be ready in about 5-7 minutes total time in water. Drain noodles and rinse in cold water until cool. Drain again.
- To serve, divide the lettuce and rice noodles into 6 bowls, lettuce on the bottom. Top with some chicken, blanched bean sprouts, shredded carrots, cucumber, scallion greens, and several spearmint and cilantro leaves. Drizzle each serving with 1 tablespoon of salad dressing and top with chopped peanuts.

Servings: 6

Tips: Choose a fish sauce with 700mg of sodium or less per tablespoon such as Tiparos brand, available at Asian markets. Due to the risk of Salmonella from eating raw sprouts, the FDA recommends that bean sprouts be blanched before consuming. Bring 4 cups of water and ½ teaspoon of salt to a rolling boil. Add sprouts and stir. Boil 30 seconds. Drain and immediately plunge sprouts into a water and ice bath. When cool, drain and spin dry.

Substitutions: Substitute 5 tablespoons reduced sodium soy sauce and 3 tablespoons of water for the fish sauce. The taste will be different but appropriately salty.

Variations: Peeled, uncooked medium shrimp can be substituted for chicken in this recipe.

Nutrition (per serving): 405 calories, 48.6g carbohydrates, 30.8g protein, 9.7g total fat, 708.3mg sodium, 3.6g fiber, 73.9mg calcium.

Chicken Stir-Fried Rice

The success of fried rice depends on using cooked but cold rice, so make rice up to 3 days ahead of time and chill. Prep the chicken and vegetables before you begin cooking, as the stir-fry goes together quickly, about 15 minutes. The total prep and cooking time is faster than calling your favorite Chinese restaurant and stopping to pick it up.

Sauce:
2 tablespoons reduced-sodium soy sauce
2 tablespoons oyster sauce
1 tablespoon rice vinegar
1 teaspoon toasted sesame oil
Stir-fry:
6 teaspoons garlic-infused oil, divided
12 ounces boneless skinless chicken breasts, cut into ½ x ¼-inch pieces
½ cup peeled, ⅓-inch diced rutabaga
½ large red bell pepper, seeded and diced into ¼-inch pieces
1 cup ½-inch pieces green beans
1 large carrot, peeled, sliced into ⅛-inch thick rounds
1 tablespoon peeled, finely chopped ginger root
4 cups cold cooked brown or white rice
2 large eggs, lightly beaten
4 scallions, green part only, thinly sliced

Substitutions: Cider vinegar can be used instead of rice vinegar. Canned, drained water chestnuts can be used in place of rutabaga. Shrimp or pork can be used in place of chicken.

Variations: For a vegetarian version, substitute cubed firm or extra-firm tofu or tempeh for meat.

Time savers: Use extra-lean ground beef or pork, no chopping required.

Nutrition (per serving): 227 calories, 27.8g carbohydrates, 14.5g protein, 6.6g total fat, 328mg sodium, 3g fiber, 41mg calcium.

- Combine the soy sauce, oyster sauce, rice vinegar, and sesame oil in a small bowl and set aside.
- Heat 2 teaspoons of garlic-infused oil in a skillet or wok on medium-high heat. Transfer chicken pieces to the pan and stir-fry until cooked through, about 3 minutes. Remove chicken to a medium bowl.
- Add 2 more teaspoons oil to skillet, then stir-fry rutabaga until it turns brown in spots. Add red bell pepper, green beans, carrots, and ginger and stir. Let vegetables rest undisturbed to allow pieces to brown. Repeat stirring vegetables with resting for 3-4 minutes. Transfer vegetables to the bowl with chicken.
- Turn heat to high and add remaining 2 teaspoons oil to coat pan. Spread the cold rice across the pan and let sit without stirring until rice starts to turn golden brown, 2-3 minutes. Stir rice and repeat process of letting rice rest and stirring until rice is golden several more times. Lower the heat to medium and push rice to one side of the pan. Pour eggs into the empty side of the pan and let sit a minute until they start to set. With a fork, gently scramble the eggs in place until completely cooked. Chop egg into small pieces and mix eggs and rice together.
- Return the cooked chicken and vegetables to the pan along with scallion greens and stir to combine. Pour sauce over mixture and stir several times, until heated through.

Servings: 8

Sweet Potato-Chard Spanish Tortilla

A Spanish omelet, called a tortilla, is typically made with white potatoes cooked slowly in a whole cup of oil. For a healthier version, sweet potatoes and Swiss chard are used, and the oil and cooking time are drastically reduced. The tortilla can be served for breakfast, lunch, dinner, or as an appetizer. Try the tortilla with Romesco Sauce (page 98).

1 medium-large sweet potato (10 ounces), peeled
1 medium-large russet potato (10 ounces), peeled
¼ cup olive oil
4 white scallion bulbs
4 scallions, green part only, thinly sliced, divided
5 cups thinly sliced Swiss chard leaves
1 teaspoon salt, divided
10 large eggs
¼ teaspoon black pepper

- Preheat broiler. Move oven rack one position below the top.
- Cut potato into ½-inch thick slices. Set aside.
- Heat oil on medium-high heat in a 10-inch, oven-proof skillet with a cover. Simmer white portion of scallion in the hot oil for 3 minutes, stirring occasionally. Remove and discard white scallion pieces. Remove 2 tablespoons of scallion-infused oil from pan and set aside.
- Transfer potato slices to skillet, add half of the scallion greens, ¾ teaspoon salt, and stir. Add ⅓ cup water, cover, and turn heat to medium-low. Cook until potatoes are softened, but still somewhat underdone, about 10 minutes, stirring halfway. Stir in chard, cover, and simmer until potatoes are soft, but very slightly firm, 4-5 minutes. Scrape potatoes and chard into a large bowl.
- Beat eggs in a medium bowl along with the remaining green part of scallions, ¼ teaspoon salt, and pepper.
- Wipe skillet clean. Add remaining 2 tablespoons of scallion-infused oil to skillet on medium-low, and coat bottom and sides of pan. Pour eggs into the bowl of sweet potatoes and chard and stir gently.
- Pour egg, potato, and chard mixture into the skillet. Cook until edges of tortilla are firm and the bottom is cooked, about 8 minutes. The middle of the tortilla will not be cooked. Put skillet under the broiler and cook just until set, 3-5 minutes. Cut into wedges and serve. Tortilla is often served slightly warm or at room temperature.

Servings: 6

Tips: For a fancier presentation, place a large serving plate or cutting board over pan before cutting the tortilla into wedges. Turn skillet and plate together, inverting tortilla onto the plate, then cut.

Substitutions: White potatoes can be used in place of sweet potatoes.

Variations: Cut tortilla into bite-sized squares and serve at room temperature as an appetizer.

Nutrition (per serving): 295 calories, 23g carbohydrates, 13.1g protein, 17.4g total fat, 597.8mg sodium, 3g fiber, 79.8mg calcium.

Baked Salmon with Herbed Cheese Sauce

This recipe is similar to one that Lisa's mother made years ago when she wanted the kids to eat fish, and it worked. A generation and a few changes later, it has succeeded with Lisa's children. This topping can be used on any fish.

1 ½ pounds salmon fillet
⅓ cup mayonnaise
1 ½ teaspoons Dijon mustard
3 tablespoons minced scallion, green part only
⅓ cup finely grated Parmesan or Romano cheese
1 teaspoon dried tarragon
1 tablespoon fresh lemon juice
⅛ teaspoon salt
Several grinds black pepper

Substitutions: 1 tablespoon fresh tarragon or other herbs can be used in place of dried. Fresh chives can be used in place of scallion greens.

Nutrition (per serving): 258 calories, 1.9g carbohydrates, 22.5g protein, 17.3g total fat, 310.8mg sodium, <1g fiber, 82.2mg calcium.

- Preheat oven to 425° F. Line a baking sheet with foil.
- Combine mayonnaise, mustard, scallion greens, cheese, tarragon, and lemon juice in a small bowl. Place salmon on a foil-lined baking sheet. Sprinkle fish lightly with salt and pepper. Coat the top of fish evenly with the sauce. Bake in the upper third of the oven until sauce is bubbling, golden brown in spots, and fish flakes when a fork is inserted, 15-20 minutes. If the fish is done and the topping isn't browned, turn oven to broil and cook until it turns golden brown, 1-2 minutes.

Servings: 6

Beef Fajitas

These have all the flavor of the fajitas you get at a Mexican restaurant. Fajitas pair well with 10-Minute Salsa (page 130) and Lime Cabbage Slaw (page 111). Marinate the steak all day for the best flavor and tenderness.

1 tablespoon ancho or New Mexico chile powder
1 teaspoon regular or smoked paprika
3 tablespoons plus 2 teaspoons garlic-infused oil, divided
¾ teaspoon salt, divided
¼ teaspoon ground black pepper
¼ cup fresh lime juice
1 ½ pounds flank, skirt or sirloin steak
8 soft corn tortillas
2 red bell peppers, seeded and sliced into long, thin strips
⅓ cup thinly sliced scallion, green part only
¼ cup sour cream
1 cup shredded cheddar cheese

- Combine cumin, ancho chile powder, smoked paprika, 2 tablespoons of olive oil, ½ teaspoon salt, pepper, and lime juice in a 2-quart zip-top bag. Add steak, remove excess air, and zip closed. Marinate meat for at least 1 hour or up to 10 hours. Heat the remaining 2 teaspoons garlic-infused oil in a large skillet on medium-high heat. Sauté bell peppers and ¼ teaspoon salt in the oil until soft and turning dark brown in spots, about 5 minutes. Add scallion greens and stir-fry for 30 seconds. Remove peppers from pan into a bowl.
- Grill or broil steak, basting with marinade to desired degree of doneness. Let meat sit 5 minutes. Slice beef across the grain at a 45 degree angle into thin strips.
- To serve fajitas: place beef strips, sour cream, sautéed red peppers, cheese, 10 Minute Salsa (page 130), Lime Cabbage Slaw (page 111), and warm tortillas in the middle of the table. Add fillings of choice to tortilla, fold in half, and enjoy with lots of napkins!

Servings: 4

Tips: There are several methods to warm soft corn tortillas so they are pliable and bend without cracking. *Microwave:* Stack tortillas on a microwave safe-plate and invert a second plate or a damp towel over the tortillas. Microwave on high power for 45-90 seconds. *Oven:* Heat oven to 350° F. Lightly pat every other tortilla with water, stack and tightly wrap in foil. Bake directly on oven rack for 10-15 minutes. *Skillet:* Heat a skillet on medium-high heat. Brush both sides of tortilla with water until damp. Cook each side, about 15 seconds, until dry but soft. Stack and keep covered.

Substitutions: If you have made the homemade Chili Powder Mix (page 125), omit individual spices and use 2 ½ tablespoons chili powder mixed with lime juice and olive oil.

Time savers: No time to make salsa or slaw? Simply top with chopped tomatoes and shredded lettuce or cabbage.

Nutrition (per serving): 611 calories, 32.2g carbohydrates, 49.4g protein, 32.3g total fat, 474.7mg sodium, 5.2g fiber, 363.7mg calcium.

Millet Stuffed Red Pepper Boats

Slice the bell peppers through the stem lengthwise to resemble boats, instead of just slicing off the tops. In addition to making a smaller serving size, the pepper halves sit stably in the pan and are easy to fill.

1 cup canned tomato puree or sauce
2 ⅔ cups water, divided
¾ teaspoon salt, divided
2 teaspoons garlic-infused oil
1 carrot, peeled, finely chopped
4 scallions, green part only, thinly sliced
1 pound extra-lean ground beef
¾ cup uncooked millet
1 ½ teaspoons dried basil
1 teaspoon dried oregano
¼ teaspoon black pepper
4 medium bell peppers (red, yellow, green, or
    orange), halved lengthwise through stem,
    seeds and stems removed
1 cup shredded sharp cheddar (4 ounces)

Tips: If you are unable to buy at least 90% lean ground beef, drain the fat from browned meat before proceeding with the recipe. You can make the filling and par-cook the peppers in advance. Fill peppers and refrigerate covered. Add a few more minutes of baking time.

Substitutions: 1 ½ cups leftover cooked brown rice, white rice, or quinoa can be used in place of millet. Omit 1 ⅔ cup water for cooking grain.

Nutrition (per serving): 242 calories, 19.7g carbohydrates, 13.7g protein, 11.8g total fat, 308.1mg sodium, 3.6g fiber, 25.7mg calcium.

- Preheat oven to 400° F. Coat both a 9 x 13-inch baking dish and 15-inch length of aluminum foil with baking spray or oil.
- Combine 1 cup tomato puree, 1 cup water, and ¼ teaspoon salt in a small bowl and set aside.
- Heat oil on medium-high heat in a large saucepan. Stir in carrots and scallion greens and cook until soft, about 4 minutes. Add ground beef and stir, chopping up meat until brown and crumbled. Pour in 1 cup diluted tomato puree, millet, basil, oregano, ½ teaspoon salt, and remaining 1 ⅔ cups water. Cover, bring to a boil, and reduce heat to a simmer. Cook until water is absorbed and millet is soft, about 25 minutes. Remove from heat.
- While filling is cooking, place peppers, cut side down, in a large Dutch oven or soup kettle. Pour in cold water to a ¼-inch depth, add ¼ teaspoon salt, cover, and bring to a boil. Reduce heat to a simmer and cook until a sharp knife inserts easily but peppers are still slightly firm, 7-10 minutes. Drain.
- Stuff peppers with filling, mounding slightly, and place in baking dish. Pour remaining 1 cup diluted tomato puree over and around peppers. Cover with foil, sprayed side down, and bake, 25-30 minutes. Uncover pan, top with cheese, and broil until cheese is melted. Serve immediately.

Servings: 8

Tips for success with low-FODMAP pastas
1. Use plenty of water in the pot to keep pasta from sticking to itself.
2. Start testing pasta to see if it is done several minutes before package directions suggest; it is easy to overcook alternative pastas, and directions are often poorly written.
3. Low-FODMAP pastas are best when freshly cooked and served immediately. Don't expect the texture to the be same the next day; however, warming up briefly in the microwave will restore some texture.

Oven-Roasted Tomato Sauce with Spaghetti and Breadcrumbs

A slow-cooked sauce tastes great; however, this simple sauce can be made on a week night from pantry ingredients. Even if you don't like anchovies, try them in this recipe where they melt away and leave behind great flavor. This sauce is a great dip for Oven-Baked Polenta Fries (page 110) or can be used any time a tomato sauce is called for in a recipe. Adapted from *Bon Appétit.*

3 tablespoons garlic-infused oil
2 anchovy filets, packed in oil
1 28-ounce can peeled whole tomatoes
3 scallions, green part only, thinly sliced
1 teaspoon dried basil
½ teaspoon dried oregano
½ teaspoon sugar
¼ teaspoon salt
⅛ teaspoon ground black pepper
½ teaspoon red pepper flakes (optional)
12 ounces low-FODMAP spaghetti (rice, corn, or quinoa)
½ cup Oven-Baked Breadcrumbs (page 130)
⅓ cup grated Parmesan cheese (1 ¼ ounce)

Tips: Double or triple recipe for extra to freeze; use extra pans to spread out the tomatoes if doubling the recipe. Freeze leftover anchovies; line a small plate with plastic wrap. Separate anchovy filets and place flat on plastic wrap and freeze. When frozen, fold wrap over and place in a zip-top bag. Frozen anchovies keep for several months.

Nutrition (per serving): 524 calories, 95g carbohydrates, 11.5g protein, 9.9g total fat, 329.4mg sodium, 2.8g fiber, 94.9mg calcium.

- Preheat oven to 425° F. Pour garlic-infused oil into a 9 x 13-inch baking pan to coat. Add anchovies and mash with a fork until pureed. Add tomatoes and their juices, scallion greens, basil, oregano, sugar, salt, pepper, and red pepper flakes. Use a small knife to cut a 1-inch slit in each tomato. Crush tomatoes with a potato masher or fork into a chunky sauce. Roast tomatoes in the middle of the oven, stirring a couple of times until sauce darkens and reduces to a jam-like consistency, 35-45 minutes. Remove pan from oven and mash tomatoes again, or puree in a food processor if you prefer a smooth sauce.
- While tomatoes are roasting, cook pasta in a large pot filled with salted water, stirring just after adding pasta and once during cooking. Boil until al dente. When pasta is nearly done, scoop out ½ cup pasta water and set aside. Drain pasta, return to pot, and toss with roasted tomato sauce. Add a few tablespoons of pasta cooking water if needed to thin sauce. Top each serving with 2 tablespoons breadcrumbs and grated Parmesan cheese.

Servings: 6

Oven-Fried Coconut Shrimp

These oven-fried crunchy coconut shrimp taste downright tropical! Serve with Orange Maple Dipping Sauce (page 126) or Pineapple Salsa (page 88).

> 1 ½ **pounds raw medium shrimp, peeled and deveined**
> ½ **cup Low-FODMAP All-Purpose Flour (page 57) or brown rice flour**
> ¾ **teaspoon salt, divided**
> 1 ½ **teaspoons curry powder, divided**
> 2 **large egg whites**
> 1 **cup unsweetened coconut flakes**
> ¾ **cup corn flake crumbs**

- Preheat oven to 400° F. Coat large baking sheet with baking spray or oil.
- Set up a breading station with 3 wide shallow dishes or bowls in order as follows:
    1. Flour: Combine flour, ⅓ teaspoon salt, and 1 teaspoon curry powder
    2. Egg whites: Beat egg whites with 2 tablespoons of water and a pinch of salt
    3. Crumbs: Combine coconut flakes, corn flake crumbs, ¼ teaspoon salt, and remaining ½ teaspoon curry powder
- Keep one dry hand at all times and one wet hand when breading the shrimp. With dry hand, place several shrimp in flour, turning to coat on all sides. With wet hand dip shrimp in egg, coating all sides, and let excess egg drip off. Place shrimp in coconut crumb mixture and use dry hand to press coconut crumbs onto shrimp to adhere. Place shrimp on the baking sheet. Bake about 15 minutes or until crust is golden.

Servings: 5

Substitutions: Corn flake crumbs can be used in place of the coconut flakes. Chicken or mild white fish, cut into strips, can be used in place of shrimp. Cornmeal can be used in place of the corn flake crumbs.

Nutrition (per serving): 338 calories, 23.2g carbohydrates, 31.9g protein, 13.1g total fat, 521.1mg sodium, 3.4g fiber, 88.3mg calcium.

Pineapple Salsa

This salsa is a great topping for fish, chicken, or pork.

> ¾ **cup diced, fresh pineapple**
> ½ **cup finely diced red bell pepper**
> 2 **scallions, green part only, thinly sliced**
> 1 **teaspoon garlic-infused oil**
> **Pinch of salt**

- Mix ingredients together and let sit for 10-15 minutes. Salsa can be made up to one day in advance and stored in the refrigerator until serving.

Servings: 5

Substitutions: Crushed, drained, canned pineapple in its own juice can be used in place of fresh pineapple. Two tablespoons finely minced chives can be used in place of scallion greens.

Nutrition (per serving): 33 calories, 5.5g carbohydrates, <1g protein, 1.2g total fat, 74mg sodium, 1g fiber, 9mg calcium.

Selecting ingredients for low-FODMAP recipes
Check the ingredients when purchasing items called for in our recipes. If they are not low FODMAP the resulting recipe won't be either. For the cheesecake, the cream cheese must not contain inulin, the lemon curd and jelly must not contain high-fructose corn syrup, and so on. See page 21 and 22 for label reading tips.

Fish Tacos with Chipotle Cream

Fish tacos are popular on restaurant menus, and now you can make them at home! They are naturally low in FODMAPs. Any mild white fish can be used in place of tilapia. Serve this recipe with Pineapple Salsa (preceding page).

Tacos:
1 ¼ pounds tilapia fillets, cut lengthwise into 1-inch wide strips
2 tablespoons extra virgin olive oil
2 tablespoons ancho chile powder
2 teaspoons ground cumin
2 teaspoons smoked paprika
½ teaspoon salt, divided
Several grinds black pepper
⅔ cup cornmeal or finely crushed corn flake crumbs
4 radishes, thinly sliced (optional)
2 cups shredded Romaine lettuce or cabbage
8 soft corn tortillas
Chipotle Cream:
½ of one canned chipotle chile pepper in adobo sauce
¼ cup mayonnaise
2 teaspoons fresh lime juice

- Preheat oven to 450° F. Line a baking sheet with foil and coat with baking spray or oil.
- Combine 2 tablespoons olive oil, chile powder, cumin, smoked paprika, ¼ teaspoon salt, and pepper in a small bowl to create a spice paste. Use a brush to coat fish fillets on both sides with the paste.
- Place cornmeal, remaining ¼ teaspoon salt, and several grinds of pepper in a shallow wide bowl or plate. Roll spiced fish pieces in cornmeal to coat and place on baking sheet. Bake until golden brown on the bottom, 6-8 minutes. Turn pieces over and bake an additional 6-9 minutes until fish is golden brown and flakes easily when a knife is inserted.
- While fish is baking prepare the Chipotle Cream. Place chipotle pepper in a small bowl and mash into a puree. Add mayonnaise, lime juice and 1-2 tablespoons of water to make a thin, pourable sauce.
- Just before serving, warm tortillas until pliable (see tips, page 85).
- To serve tacos, place fish in warmed tortilla, drizzle with chipotle cream, add sliced radishes and lettuce.

Servings: 4

Tips: Chipotle cream can be made several days in advance and held in the refrigerator. Chipotles in adobo sauce are sold in a small can. Note the recipe calls for half a pepper, not half a can! Leftover chiles can be frozen.

Substitutions: ½ teaspoon ground chipotle chile powder can be used in place of chipotle chile pepper.

Time savers: Two tablespoons of Chili Powder Mix (page 125) can be used in place of the ancho chile powder, cumin, and paprika in the spice paste. The cornmeal adds a crunchy texture, but you can skip this step to save time and bake the fish with spice paste only. Double recipe and, before cooking, freeze half of the fish pieces on a baking sheet lined with foil. Once frozen, pop breaded fish into a zip-top bag. Cook fish frozen, but lower oven temperature to 350° F and bake a few minutes more.

Nutrition (per serving): 439 calories, 41.3g carbohydrates, 33.9g protein, 16.9g total fat, 464.7mg sodium, 6.1g fiber, 137.5mg calcium.

Chicken Nuggets with Maple Mustard Dipping Sauce

This family-friendly meal is enjoyed by kids and adults alike. Baking nuggets on a cooling rack means very little oil is used, they get crispy all over, and little attention is needed when cooking.

Chicken nuggets:
1 ½ pounds boneless, skinless chicken breast
¾ cup brown rice flour or Low-FODMAP All-
     Purpose Flour (page 57)
½ teaspoon salt, divided
½ teaspoon ground black pepper, divided
¼ teaspoon asafetida (optional)
2 large eggs
2 tablespoons Dijon mustard
2 cups coarsely crushed corn flake crumbs (about
     6 ½ cups uncrushed)
2 teaspoons basil
½ teaspoon oregano
½ teaspoon paprika
Maple Mustard Dipping Sauce
3 tablespoons 100% pure maple syrup
2 tablespoons Dijon mustard
2 tablespoons mayonnaise

- Preheat oven to 400° F. Line a large baking sheet with foil. Place a wire cooling rack on top of foil and coat rack with baking spray or oil.
- Set up a breading station with 3 shallow dishes or pans (pie or cake pans work well).
    1. Flour: Mix flour, ¼ teaspoon salt, ¼ teaspoon black pepper, and asafetida
    2. Eggs: Beat eggs, Dijon mustard, and 1 tablespoon water
    3. Crumbs: Mix corn flake crumbs, basil, oregano, paprika, ¼ teaspoon salt, and ¼ teaspoon pepper
- Cut chicken breasts lengthwise into ½-inch thick strips. Cut strips crosswise into equal pieces, 3-4 inches long. Place half of the chicken strips into flour in Dish 1 and toss pieces to coat with flour. Use a fork to transfer 1-2 pieces into egg mixture in Dish 2 and coat pieces all over with egg. Lift pieces from egg with a fork, letting excess egg drip off. Place chicken strips into corn flake crumbs in Dish 3. Coat with crumbs on all sides, pressing to adhere, and transfer to oiled rack. Repeat the process with the remaining chicken.
- Coat the tops of the strips with baking spray or oil. Bake in the middle of the oven until golden and crisp, 25-30 minutes.
- Stir dipping sauce ingredients together in a small bowl and serve with the chicken nuggets.

Servings: 5

Tips: To make corn flake crumbs, place corn flakes in a gallon zip-top bag and close bag, leaving a tiny opening. Crush corn flakes coarsely with a rolling pin or the bottom of a saucepan until pieces are the size of sesame seeds; coarser pieces makes crunchier nuggets. If a cooling rack is not available, you can bake the chicken directly on the foil; grease the foil well and turn pieces over about halfway through baking.

Substitutions: Low-FODMAP bread crumbs or cornmeal can be used in place of corn flake crumbs.

Variations: For Mexican chicken nuggets, add 1 ½ teaspoons Chili Powder Mix (page 125) each to flour in Dish 1 and to corn flake crumbs in Dish 3; serve with 10 Minute Salsa (page 130). Or use 1 ½ teaspoon Barbecue Spice Rub (page 125) and serve with Barbecue Sauce (page 101).

Nutrition (per serving): 224 calories, 34.7g carbohydrates, 10.2g protein, 5.2g total fat, 601.7mg sodium, 1.7g fiber, 35.1mg calcium.

Eggplant Puttanesca

This spicy sauce can be served on Microwave Polenta (page 110), crispy, fried polenta, pasta, or pizza crust.

2 tablespoons garlic-infused oil
1 medium unpeeled eggplant (1-1 ¼ pounds),
    diced into ½-inch pieces
½ red bell pepper, seeded and diced
2 large tomatoes, diced into ¼-inch pieces
2 teaspoons dried basil
1 teaspoon oregano
½ teaspoon salt
4 scallions, green part only, finely sliced
10 Kalamata olives, pitted and sliced
1 tablespoon capers
½ teaspoon red pepper flakes (optional)
½ cup water

Nutrition (per serving): 114 calories, 11g carbohydrates, 2.1g protein, 7.8g total fat, 411.1mg sodium, 5g fiber, 43mg calcium.

- Heat 1 tablespoon oil in a sauté pan or large skillet on medium-high heat. Distribute diced eggplant across the pan, stir, and let sit without moving pieces until they turn brown on the bottom, about 4 minutes. Add remaining tablespoon oil and bell pepper and stir, turning eggplant pieces to brown on another side, about 3 minutes. Stir in remaining ingredients. Reduce heat and simmer, stirring periodically until sauce is thick and eggplant is soft, about 15 minutes. Add a few tablespoons of water if sauce starts to stick to the bottom of the pot before eggplant is done. Serve immediately.

Servings: 5

Grilled Herbed Lemon Chicken

Serve on top of a salad along with a cooked grain (quinoa, rice), and pumpkin seeds or toasted walnuts for a complete meal.

2 pounds boneless, skinless chicken thighs (or
    breasts)
¼ cup fresh lemon juice
¼ cup garlic-infused oil
2 teaspoons granulated sugar
2 tablespoons chopped fresh rosemary
1 tablespoon fresh thyme leaves
2 tablespoons fresh oregano
⅓ cup minced scallions, green part only
1 teaspoon lemon zest
½ teaspoon salt
½ teaspoon ground black pepper

Time savers: If you have Lemon Vinaigrette (page 129) already made, use ½ cup in place of the lemon juice, oil, and sugar.

Substitutions: If fresh herbs aren't available, substitute 2 teaspoons dried, crushed rosemary, 1 teaspoon dried thyme and 2 teaspoons dried oregano.

Nutrition (per serving): 68 calories, 1.6g carbohydrates, 2.8g protein, 5.7g total fat, 106.4mg sodium, <1g fiber, 10.9mg calcium.

- Cut each chicken thigh into three pieces of uniform size. Combine lemon juice, oil, sugar, herbs, lemon zest, salt, and pepper in a gallon zip-top bag. Add chicken pieces, close bag, and remove as much air as possible. Marinate for at least 1 hour or up to 12 hours. Grill or broil, basting with marinade while cooking to an internal temperature of 165° F.

Servings: 6

Enchiladas

Vary the amount of enchilada sauce you use in this recipe to suit yourself.

> 2 teaspoons garlic-infused oil
> 1 lb extra-lean ground beef, turkey, or chicken
> ¼ teaspoon salt
> 2 scallions, green part only, thinly sliced
> 4 ½ cups enchilada sauce, divided (below)
> 12 soft corn tortillas, warmed until pliable (see
>   tips, page 85)
> 1 cup shredded extra sharp cheddar cheese (4
>   ounces)

- Preheat oven to 375° F. Coat a 9 x 13-inch baking pan with baking spray or oil.
- Heat garlic-infused oil in a skillet over medium-high heat. Add beef and salt and sauté, breaking up meat until no longer pink. Stir in scallion greens and 1 cup enchilada sauce and cook 1 minute.
- Spread ½ cup enchilada sauce over the bottom of the baking pan. Place tortilla on a flat surface and fill with 3 tablespoons meat mixture in the center. Fold each side of the tortilla around the filling and place seam side down in prepared pan. Repeat until all tortillas are filled.
- Pour 3 cups enchilada sauce over top of the enchiladas. Sprinkle cheese over the top and bake until bubbling and heated through, about 20 minutes.

Servings: 6

Tips: If you are unable to buy at least 90% lean ground meat or poultry, drain the browned meat before proceeding with the recipe.

Substitutions: Cooked pork, beef or chicken, can be used in place of ground meat.

Time savers: Supermarket rotisserie chicken (pre-cooked) can be used.

Nutrition (per serving): 499 calories, 36.3g carbohydrates, 22.8g protein, 30.6g total fat, 1023.7mg sodium, 6.4g fiber, 250.8mg calcium.

Enchilada Sauce

This mild enchilada sauce uses ancho chile powder which is just ground ancho chile pods, with no other additives.

> 3 tablespoons ground ancho or New Mexico chile
>   powder
> 1 tablespoon ground cumin
> ½ teaspoon smoked paprika
> 1 ½ tablespoons brown rice or sorghum flour
> 1 teaspoon salt
> ¼ teaspoon ground black pepper
> 1 teaspoon unsweetened cocoa powder (optional)
> 3 tablespoons garlic-infused oil
> ½ cup thinly sliced scallions, green part only
> 2 ½ cups water
> 1 (28-ounce) can tomato puree
> 1 ½ teaspoons granulated sugar

- Preheat oven to 375° F.
- Combine chile powder, cumin, smoked paprika, flour, salt, pepper, and cocoa powder in a small bowl and set aside.
- Heat garlic-infused oil on medium-high heat in a 2-quart saucepan. Add scallion greens and sauté for 1 minute. Add spice mixture to pan and stir continuously until spices smell fragrant, 30-60 seconds. Pour 2 ½ cups of water into the spice mixture slowly, while stirring, until mixture is smooth and no lumps remain. Stir in tomato puree and sugar until smooth. Bring to a simmer and cook uncovered for 20 minutes, stirring periodically. Serve immediately or refrigerate for up to four days.

Servings: 10, ½ cup each. **Yield:** 5 cups

Tips: Use extra Enchilada Sauce on your enchiladas, tacos, quesadillas, chicken, etc. It also freezes well.

Substitutions: If you have made Chili Powder Mix (page 125), you can use 4 tablespoons in place of the ancho, cumin, and paprika.

Nutrition (per serving): 69 calories, 7.1g carbohydrates, 1.3g protein, 4.8g total fat, 370.4mg sodium, 2.1g fiber, 40.8mg calcium.

Pad Thai

Cranberry juice's sweet, tart taste makes a great substitute for the tamarind juice traditionally used in this dish, as it is FODMAP-friendly and easy to find. Have all of the food prepped in advance; the cooking process goes quickly.

¾ cup sugar-sweetened cranberry juice (no high-fructose corn syrup or fruit juice blends)
¼ cup packed light brown sugar
½ cup water
¼ cup fish sauce
½ teaspoon salt
1 pound uncooked Asian rice noodles, ¼-inch thick
2 tablespoons garlic-infused oil, divided
¾ pound boneless skinless chicken breasts, cut into 1- by ½-inch pieces
1 cup peeled, chopped rutabaga (¼ pound), cut into 1- by ¼-inch pieces
½ red bell pepper, seeded and chopped into ½-inch pieces
1 ½ cups thinly shredded green cabbage
1 ½ cups mung bean sprouts (6 ounces)
2 large eggs, lightly beaten
4 scallions, green part only, thinly sliced
½ cup coarsely chopped roasted peanuts

Tips: Choose a fish sauce with 700mg of sodium or less per tablespoon such as Tiparos brand, available at Asian markets. If you prefer a sweeter sauce, use up to ½ cup brown sugar. Sauce can be made several days in advance.

Substitutions: Raw, peeled shrimp or cubed tempeh or tofu can be used in place of chicken. Thinly sliced bok choy or Swiss chard can be used in place of cabbage.

Nutrition (per serving): 553 calories, 85g carbohydrates, 22.7g protein, 13.5g total fat, 1410.8mg sodium, 4g fiber, 84.2mg calcium.

- Combine the cranberry juice, brown sugar, water, fish sauce, and salt in a wide, deep skillet. Turn heat to medium-high and bring to a boil, stirring until sugar dissolves. Turn heat down and simmer until sauce is thick and syrupy and is reduced to 1 cup, 6-8 minutes. Remove from heat and set aside.
- Bring a large pot of water to a boil. Add rice noodles. Boil 2 minutes, stirring to break up noodle bundle. Remove from heat, stir again, and let sit for 2 more minutes. Test a strand. Noodles are ready to drain when they are softened but still slightly underdone and firm in the center. They will be cooked further in the stir-fry. Drain noodles and set aside.
- In a large wok, heat 1 tablespoon oil. Have a medium bowl nearby. Add chicken or shrimp to wok. Stir-fry until cooked through. Remove cooked chicken or shrimp to the bowl and set aside. Add 2 teaspoons of oil and heat for 30 seconds, then stir-fry rutabaga until pieces soften, 1-2 minutes. Add red bell pepper and fry 1 minute. Add cabbage and stir until soft, 2 minutes. Add bean sprouts and stir-fry 1 minute. Clear the center of the pan by pushing vegetables to the sides. Add 1 teaspoon of oil to the center and pour in eggs. Cook eggs without stirring until they begin to set. Scramble eggs slightly in the center of the pan, keeping vegetables at the edge. Continue lightly scrambling eggs until completely cooked. Chop eggs into small pieces and stir to combine with the vegetables. Return chicken or shrimp to pan, then add noodles and pour sauce evenly over the food. Add ¼ cup of water to pan and toss noodles gently with the ingredients until they are soft and have absorbed all the liquid, 3-4 minutes. Test a noodle and if not done, add several tablespoons of water and continue tossing mixture until noodles are soft. Stir in scallion greens, remove from heat, and sprinkle with peanuts.

Servings: 6

Skillet Hamburger and Elbows

This one-pot meal is comfort food for the whole family. For a grown-up version, use stronger cheeses like extra-sharp cheddar, Parmesan, Romano, Asiago, or Gouda.

2 teaspoons paprika
½ teaspoon smoked paprika
1 teaspoon dry mustard powder
1 teaspoon ancho chile powder
1 teaspoon oregano
1 teaspoon salt
¼ teaspoon ground black pepper
1 pound extra-lean ground beef
1 tablespoon garlic-infused oil
½ red bell pepper, seeded and finely chopped
4 scallions, green part only, thinly sliced
2 cups lactose-free milk
1 medium tomato, finely chopped
1 tablespoon reduced-sodium soy sauce
2 ½ cups uncooked low-FODMAP elbow
    macaroni (rice, quinoa, or corn)
1 cup chopped fresh green beans
1 tablespoon cornstarch dissolved in 2
    tablespoons cold water
1 ¼ cups shredded sharp cheese (5 ounces)

Tips: If you are unable to buy at least 90% lean ground beef, drain the browned meat before proceeding with the recipe.

Substitutions: 1 tablespoon of prepared mustard can be used in place of 1 teaspoon dry mustard. Finely diced yellow squash or zucchini can be used instead of green beans.

Nutrition (per serving): 493 calories, 41.5g carbohydrates, 23.8g protein, 24.8g total fat, 756.3mg sodium, 4.5g fiber, 292.5mg calcium.

- Combine paprika, smoked paprika, dry mustard, chile powder, oregano, salt, and pepper in a small bowl and set aside.
- Heat oil in a large sauté pan or Dutch oven on medium-high. Add hamburger, stirring to break up meat. Let meat brown well before stirring. When meat is nearly done, stir in red bell pepper and scallion greens and continue cooking until meat is no longer pink. Stir in milk, 2 cups water, tomato, soy sauce, spice mix, and uncooked pasta. Cover pan and bring to a boil, then reduce heat to a simmer. Cook covered until pasta is slightly underdone, about 4 minutes less than the recommended cooking time. Stir in green beans, then cornstarch mixture. Cover and cook until pasta is done, 4 minutes. Remove cover, add cheese, and stir until cheese melts into the sauce. Turn off heat and let dish sit for a minute or two to allow it to thicken.

Servings: 6

Korean Barbecued Beef

This marinade uses kiwi as a meat tenderizer, and tastes similar to teriyaki. Serve Korean Barbecued Beef over warm, short-grain rice.

3 pounds rib eye beef cut across the grain into
    thin strips (3 x ½ x ⅛-inch thick)
3 ½ tablespoons toasted sesame oil
3 cloves garlic, peeled and very coarsely chopped
5 scallions, white part only, chopped into ¼-inch
    pieces
5 scallions, green part only, cut into 2-inch pieces
½ kiwi, peeled
3 tablespoons peeled, chopped fresh ginger root
⅓ cup light brown sugar
½ cup reduced-sodium soy sauce or tamari

Tips: To make cutting thin pieces easier, freeze meat for 30-40 minutes. Slice across the grain on a diagonal.

Substitutions: Other meat cuts can be used, including boneless short ribs, flap steak, flank steak, skirt steak, or sirloin. Granulated sugar can be used instead of brown sugar.

- Measure oil, coarsely chopped garlic cloves, and white part of scallions into to a small skillet on medium-low heat and cook until the oil bubbles and garlic turns yellow, swirling pan periodically, 3-4 minutes. Pour oil through a sieve, or remove garlic and scallion pieces with a spoon and discard.

- Place infused sesame oil, scallion greens, kiwi, ginger, brown sugar, soy sauce or tamari, and ¼ cup water in the bowl of a food processor or blender. Puree until smooth. Place sliced beef in a zip-top plastic bag and pour marinade over meat. Marinate beef for 1-4 hours. Barbecue or broil, basting with marinade, to desired level of doneness. Serve over rice.

Servings: 10

Nutrition (per serving): 372 calories, 4.7g carbohydrates, 28.5g protein, 25.9g total fat, 285.2mg sodium, <1g fiber, 21.3mg calcium.

Mac 'n Cheese with Hidden Squash

Adding grated vegetables to macaroni and cheese allows you to sneak vegetables into a dish that kids are inclined to like. The shredded summer squash virtually disappears in the sauce. The dish can be served from the stovetop, or it can be baked into a crunchy, crumb-topped casserole.

2 tablespoons cornstarch
2 ¾ cups lactose-free milk
2 tablespoons extra virgin olive oil
2 cups shredded yellow summer squash or
    zucchini (about ½ pound)
⅓ cup thinly sliced scallions, green part only
2 teaspoons dry mustard powder
¾ teaspoon salt
Several generous grinds pepper
2 cups coarsely shredded sharp cheddar cheese (8
    ounces)
½ cup shredded Parmesan or Romano cheese (2
    ounces)
1 pound low-FODMAP elbow macaroni, cooked
    (if making oven-baked casserole, under-cook
    pasta by 2-3 minutes)
½ cup coarsely crushed corn flake crumbs or
    Oven-Baked Breadcrumbs (page 130)

- Preheat oven to 400° F. Coat a 9 x 13-inch baking pan generously with baking spray or oil.
- Measure cornstarch into a medium bowl; slowly whisk in milk until cornstarch is dissolved and mixture is smooth. Heat olive oil in a Dutch oven or stockpot over medium heat. Stir milk-cornstarch mixture again and slowly add it to the oil while whisking. Bring mixture to a low simmer while whisking periodically until it thickens slightly. Add squash, scallion greens, dry mustard, salt, and pepper. Increase heat to medium-high and cook until mixture thickens even more, 3-5 minutes. Add both cheeses and stir until melted. Stir in partially cooked pasta. Pour mixture into prepared pan and top evenly with crumbs. Bake until hot and bubbling, 20-25 minutes. If topping is not golden brown, broil on top rack 2-3 minutes.

Servings: 12

Tips: Leftovers reheat easily in a microwave, or cover with foil and bake at 300° F, 20-25 minutes.

Substitutions: ¼ cup chives can be used instead of ⅓ cup scallion greens.

Variations: Omit yellow squash and add 1 ½ cup cooked, mashed kabocha or butternut squash. For a grownup version, replace cheddar with Gruyere, Fontina, Asiago, or smoked Gouda (or a combo). Add 1 teaspoon smoked paprika and a few pinches of cayenne pepper.

Time savers: Serve immediately instead of baking the casserole. Simmer an extra 2-4 minutes to finish cooking the pasta. Peeled, cubed butternut squash can be purchased in the produce department.

Nutrition (per serving): 289 calories, 37.1g carbohydrates, 8.7g protein, 11g total fat, 366.9mg sodium, 3.2g fiber, 257.5mg calcium.

Mediterranean Chicken on Roasted Potatoes

The ingredients combine to make a fragrantly spiced sauce. Mild, Spanish smoked paprika (a.k.a. Pimenton de la Vera) adds an incomparable smoky taste to foods.

1 ½ pounds red-skinned potatoes, cut into ¼-inch
    slices
¼ teaspoon salt
⅛ teaspoon ground black pepper
1 pint grape tomatoes (10 ounces)
2 tablespoons garlic-infused oil
Spice paste:
1 tablespoon lemon juice
1 teaspoon dried thyme
1½ teaspoons ground cumin
1½ teaspoons paprika or smoked paprika
½ teaspoon ground coriander seed
¼ teaspoon salt
Several generous grinds black pepper
1 ½ pounds boneless, skinless chicken breast
    halves

- Preheat oven to 475° F. Coat the bottom and sides of a 9 x 13-inch baking pan with baking spray or oil.
- Arrange sliced potatoes in two layers in the prepared baking pan, sprinkling salt and pepper over each layer. Scatter tomatoes over the potatoes. Drizzle oil over vegetables and roast on the middle rack until potatoes are soft but still slightly underdone and tomatoes are soft, about 15 minutes. While the vegetables are roasting, mix spice paste ingredients in a small bowl and set aside.
- Remove the pan from the oven. Place chicken on top of the partially roasted vegetables. Coat the top of chicken pieces with the spice paste. Return pan to the oven and roast uncovered until chicken has reached 170° F internal temperature, 20-25 minutes.

Servings: 4

Variations: Mild, white fish like cod, haddock, or tilapia can be used instead of chicken. Reduce cooking time by 5-10 minutes.

Time savers: Combine dry spices in triple amounts and store in an airtight container to use as a spice rub for future recipes.

Nutrition (per serving): 406 calories, 35.8g carbohydrates, 43.8g protein, 9.6g total fat, 275.3mg sodium, 4.2g fiber, 53mg calcium.

Orange Chicken

This fast and easy chicken dish will appeal to all ages. Serve with rice and sautéed spinach or Swiss chard.

1 ½ pounds boneless, skinless chicken thighs
1 cup Lisa's Chicken Stock (page 146) or water,
    divided
1 teaspoon cornstarch
3 tablespoons red wine vinegar
½ teaspoon salt, divided
¼ teaspoon ground black pepper
⅓ cup orange marmalade
1 tablespoon garlic-infused oil or canola oil
1 teaspoon ground coriander
2 scallions, green part only, finely sliced
1 teaspoon orange zest
1 teaspoon Dijon mustard

- Combine ½ cup chicken stock, cornstarch, vinegar, ¼ teaspoon salt, and pepper in a small bowl, stirring until cornstarch has dissolved. Stir in marmalade and set aside.
- Heat oil in a large skillet on medium-high heat. Add coriander and stir

Variations: For Asian-style chicken, omit coriander. Before adding water or chicken stock to deglaze pan, sauté 2 teaspoons minced, peeled ginger root until soft, about 1 minute. Add remaining ingredients and 2 tablespoons soy sauce.

Nutrition calculated using water (per serving): 307 calories, 19.2g carbohydrates, 33.8g protein, 10.2g total fat, 469mg sodium, <1g fiber, 37.3mg calcium.

for 30 seconds. Distribute chicken pieces in skillet, sprinkle with remaining ¼ teaspoon salt and several grinds black pepper. Cover and cook without disturbing until deep golden brown, 6-8 minutes. Turn chicken over, cover, and cook on the other side about 5 more minutes. Remove chicken to a plate and cover to keep warm. Add remaining ½ cup chicken stock to the skillet, scraping up brown bits on the bottom of the pan. Add marmalade mixture, scallion greens, and zest and stir until liquid thickens, about 1 minute. Whisk in mustard until smooth. Return chicken and juices to the skillet, cover, and simmer until chicken is cooked through and sauce is thick, about 5 minutes.

Servings: 4

Pasta Spinach Pie

This hearty one-dish meal is a crowd pleaser.

> **1 pound low-FODMAP elbows, penne, or rotini (rice, corn, or quinoa)**
> **2 teaspoons garlic-infused oil**
> **1 pound extra-lean ground turkey**
> **12 ounces baby spinach leaves**
> **8 large eggs**
> **2 ½ cups lactose-free milk**
> **1 ½ teaspoon dried basil**
> **1 teaspoon dried oregano**
> **1 tablespoon dry mustard powder**
> **1 teaspoon fennel seeds, finely chopped**
> **1 cup shredded sharp cheddar (4 ounces)**
> **½ cup shredded Romano or Parmesan cheese (2 ounces)**
> **6 scallions, green part only, finely sliced**
> **1 teaspoon salt**
> **½ teaspoon black pepper**

- Preheat oven to 350° F. Coat a 9 x 13 x 2-inch baking pan with baking spray or oil.
- Boil pasta in salted water for about ⅔ of the usual cooking time so that pasta is underdone and slightly hard in the center. Drain pasta and transfer into a large mixing bowl.
- Heat oil in a Dutch oven or large saucepan over medium-high heat. Sauté and crumble ground turkey in the oil until no longer pink. Transfer the turkey to the bowl with the pasta.
- Put spinach and 3 tablespoons of water in the saucepan. Cover and cook on medium until leaves are wilted, about 3 minutes. Drain, squeeze out excess water. Transfer the cooked spinach to the bowl of pasta and turkey.
- Beat eggs and milk in a medium bowl. Stir in basil, oregano, dry mustard, fennel seeds, cheeses, scallion greens, salt, and pepper. Pour the egg mixture over the pasta, turkey, and spinach and stir to combine. Transfer the mixture into prepared baking pan. Coat a large piece of foil with baking spray or oil and cover the casserole, oiled side down. Bake in the middle of the oven for 45 minutes. Increase oven temperature to 375° F, remove foil and bake for an additional 15 minutes until pasta pie is hot and browned in places. Cut and serve immediately.

Servings: 12

Substitutions: Ground beef can be used in place of ground turkey. If you are unable to purchase 90% lean ground turkey or beef, drain the browned meat before proceeding with the recipe. Chopped mature spinach leaves, chard, or kale can be used in place of baby spinach.

Time savers: Frozen, chopped spinach may be used; thaw, squeeze out excess water and add to the bowl with cooked ground turkey.

Nutrition (per serving): 594 calories, 78.1g carbohydrates, 29.4g protein, 17.3g total fat, 604.4mg sodium, 1.7g fiber, 377.3mg calcium.

Crispy Pan-Fried Cod with Romesco Sauce

This pan-frying technique can be used with any type of fish fillet, though cooking time may vary.

2 pounds boneless, skinless cod fillets
3 tablespoons Low-FODMAP All-Purpose Flour
(page 57) or brown rice flour
¾ teaspoon cumin
¼ teaspoon smoked paprika
¼ teaspoon salt
Several grinds black pepper
1 tablespoon butter
¾ cup Romesco Sauce (below)

Nutrition (per serving): 233 calories, 7.1g carbohydrates, 28.9g protein, 9.6g total fat, 271.7mg sodium, 1.6g fiber, 45mg calcium.

- Combine flour, spices, salt, and pepper in a shallow bowl. Roll fish in flour or dust both sides of fish with mixture placed in a sieve and tapped over fish. Heat a large skillet on medium-high heat. Melt butter. Place cod in skillet and cook without moving fish until a brown crust forms, 3-5 minutes. Gently turn fish over and cook until fish is browned and flakes easily. Serve fish topped with a spoonful of Romesco Sauce (below).

Servings: 6

Romesco Sauce

This addictive Spanish sauce is traditionally served with fish or seafood, but it also pairs well with grilled meats, and can be used as a dip for veggies or Oven-Baked Polenta Fries (page 110), or tossed into cooked potatoes or pasta. In fact, it is good on everything!

2 medium tomatoes, halved (10 ounces total)
2 medium red bell peppers, halved and seeded
¼ cup plus 2 teaspoons garlic-infused oil, divided
½ cup toasted, sliced almonds
1 slice low-FODMAP bread, toasted golden
brown, torn into pieces
1 ½ tablespoons ancho chile powder
1 teaspoon smoked paprika
½ teaspoon salt
Several generous grinds black pepper
2 tablespoons red wine vinegar

Substitutions: Whole grape or cherry tomatoes can be used instead of larger tomatoes; no need to peel them. ¼ cup low-FODMAP bread crumbs can be used in place of 1 slice of low-FODMAP bread. Any mild chile powder can be used in place of ancho. If you don't have a food processor, cut the vegetables up into smaller pieces by hand, then grind all ingredients at once in a blender to finish.

Time Saver: Two drained roasted red peppers from a jar can be used instead of broiling and peeling your own peppers. Use a 14.5-ounce can of fire-roasted tomatoes, drained.

- Cover baking sheet with foil and oil lightly. Place tomatoes cut side down on one end of the baking sheet and peppers cut side down on the other end. Press pepper down firmly with hand to flatten completely. Brush vegetables with 2 teaspoons of oil. Broil tomatoes and peppers until skin is blackened all over, removing each one from oven as it is done, 7-10 minutes. Place vegetables in a bowl and cover with plastic wrap for 10 minutes. Peel and discard charred skin from peppers and tomatoes. A few small bits left on are fine.
- Pulse almonds, toasted bread, chile powder, smoked paprika, salt, and pepper together in a food processor to form a coarse crumb. Add roasted tomatoes, bell peppers, and vinegar, and pulse to form a chunky paste. With processor running, add ¼ cup of oil in a steady stream to form a coarse paste. Do not over-process. Use within 4 days or freeze extra in ice cube trays to have ready at any time.

Nutrition (per serving): 77 calories, 3.9g carbohydrates, 1.5g protein, 6.5g total fat, 92.3mg sodium, 1.4g fiber, 17mg calcium.

Servings: 16, 2 tablespoons each. Yield: 2 cups

Noodles with Tempeh and Peanut Sauce

This dish is a good excuse to try tempeh if you have never eaten it. It is a good protein source which takes on any other flavors in a dish. The sweetness of the squash pairs well with the peanut sauce. Allow time to make the peanut sauce and prep the vegetables before starting this recipe so they will be ready when you need them.

Noodles:
1 pound uncooked Thai style rice noodles, ¼-inch
    wide (or rice, corn, or quinoa pasta)
Peanut Sauce:
2 tablespoons toasted sesame oil
2 garlic cloves, coarsely chopped
1 rounded tablespoon peeled, finely minced
    ginger
½ cup creamy peanut butter
¼ cup reduced-sodium soy sauce or tamari
2 tablespoons Lisa's Ketchup (page 126)
¼ cup packed light brown sugar
1 teaspoon red pepper flakes (optional)
1 cup water
2 tablespoons unseasoned rice vinegar
Stir-fry:
1 ½ tablespoons canola or peanut oil, divided
12 ounces tempeh, cut into ¼- x ¼- x 1-inch
    pieces
1 ½ cups peeled, chopped butternut squash
1 red bell pepper, seeded and chopped
2 ½ cups shredded green cabbage
4 scallions, green part only, thinly sliced

Tips: Peanut sauce freezes well and can be served warm or cold, so consider making a double batch. It makes a great dipping sauce for grilled chicken, chicken nuggets, or shrimp.

Substitutions: Peeled, sliced sweet potato or rutabaga can be used in place of butternut squash. Cooked rice, quinoa, or millet can be used in place of noodles.

Nutrition (per serving): 495 calories, 69.8g carbohydrates, 15.3g protein, 19.2g total fat, 456.1mg sodium, 3.8g fiber, 103.1mg calcium.

- Fill a large Dutch oven or saucepan with water and bring to a boil. Add rice noodles and boil for 2 minutes, stirring to separate noodles. Turn off heat and let noodles sit in the water for 2 more minutes. Stir and test a strand to see if it is done (chewy, but not mushy). If not, leave the noodles soaking and test a noodle every minute thereafter. Noodles are done in 5-8 minutes total time, depending on the thickness of noodles. Drain, place in a large serving bowl.
- Heat sesame oil and garlic in a small saucepan. When oil bubbles, turn to low and cook until garlic turns yellow (do not brown), about 2 minutes. Discard garlic. Add ginger to oil and stir for 30 seconds. Stir in peanut butter, soy sauce, Lisa's Ketchup (page 126), brown sugar, and red pepper flakes. Pour in 1 cup water and simmer, stirring a few times, until sauce is the texture of heavy cream, 2-3 minutes. Stir in vinegar and thin with more water if needed. Pour ⅔ of the peanut sauce over noodles and toss gently to coat. Cover noodles to keep warm and save the remaining peanut sauce for stir-fry.
- Heat 1 tablespoon canola oil in a large wok on medium-high heat. Add tempeh and stir-fry until golden and crispy with a few charred spots, 4-6 minutes. Remove tempeh to a small bowl. Add remaining ½ tablespoon oil, then briefly stir in butternut squash. Let squash sit without stirring until it browns in spots, 2 minutes. Stir and let rest another 1-2 minutes. Add red pepper, and stir-fry about 2 minutes. Add cabbage and stir-fry until wilted, about 2 minutes. Return tempeh to the wok, add scallion greens and stir to combine. Stir in remaining peanut sauce. Pour vegetable mixture over noodles and serve.

Servings: 8

Pasta with Roasted Butternut Squash and Swiss Chard

The caramelization of natural sugars in foods as it browns during roasting is a cooking trick which adds a lot of flavor. It is worth the few extra minutes of cooking time.

3 cups peeled, seeded, ½-inch cubed, butternut
    squash (1 pound)
2 tablespoons garlic-infused oil
1 teaspoon dried thyme
½ teaspoon dried sage
1 teaspoon salt, divided
Pepper
12 ounces uncooked low-FODMAP pasta (rice,
    corn, quinoa)
1 bunch Swiss chard, washed (10 ounces)
3 scallions, green part only, sliced
⅓ cup grated Parmesan or Romano cheese (1 ¼
    ounce)

- Preheat oven to 425° F. Lightly coat large baking sheet with baking spray or oil.
- Toss butternut squash with 1 tablespoon of garlic-infused oil, thyme, sage, ½ teaspoon of salt, and a few grinds of pepper. Spread squash on the prepared baking sheet in a single layer so that squash is not crowded. Roast in oven until browned, about 15 minutes. Turn pieces and continue roasting about 10 more minutes until browned on the other side. Squash should still be slightly firm. Remove from oven.
- While squash is roasting, bring a large pot of water to boil. Add pasta, reduce heat and simmer.
- Cut stems off the Swiss chard. Cut stems into ½-inch thick pieces, wash, drain, and set aside. Slice chard leaves into 1-inch wide pieces, wash, and drain. Five minutes before pasta is done, add chard stems to the pasta water. Boil 2 minutes, then add chard leaves for the last 3 minutes of cooking time. Scoop out ½ cup pasta water and set aside. Drain pasta and chard and return them to the pot. Add roasted butternut squash and herbs. Toss pasta and squash with 2 teaspoons of garlic-flavored olive oil, chopped scallion greens, cheese, ½ teaspoon of salt, several generous grinds of pepper, and some of the pasta water a few tablespoons at a time to make a sauce.

Servings: 6

Tips: A vegetable peeler does a good job of removing the thin outer layer of skin from a butternut squash. Crowding the squash in a too-small pan will cause it to steam instead of browning. If you don't have a large baking sheet, use two 9 x 13-inch baking pans instead.

Substitutions: 10 ounces of baby spinach may be used in place of chard. ⅓ cup of goat cheese can be used in place of Parmesan or Romano.

Time savers: Use peeled butternut squash, available in most produce sections.

Nutrition (per serving): 556 calories, 99.9g carbohydrates, 13.5g protein, 11.3g total fat, 614.7mg sodium, 4.5g fiber, 125.5mg calcium.

Slow Cooker Pulled Pork with Barbecue Sauce

The Barbecue Spice Rub provides that barbecue taste, even without grilling. This recipe is designed for a 6-quart slow cooker, but can be made on the stove top, too. There is plenty of time to make the Barbecue Sauce while the pork is cooking.

4 ½ pounds pork tenderloin (2 large tenderloins)
3 tablespoons Barbecue Spice Rub (page 125)
2 tablespoons garlic-infused oil
½ teaspoon salt
½ teaspoon black pepper
¼ cup cider vinegar
2 tablespoons packed light brown sugar
4 leek leaves or 6 scallions, green part only, left
    whole
½ chipotle chile in adobo sauce, finely minced
    (optional)
1 cup Barbecue Sauce (next page)

Tips: No slow cooker? Stove top directions: Brown meat in a Dutch oven or stock pot; add remaining ingredients and increase water to 2 cups. Simmer covered, until pork shreds easily, 75-90 minutes, adding more water if needed.

Substitutions: If you don't have Barbecue Spice Rub on hand, combine the following spices

- Sprinkle spice rub all over the pork and rub it on. Heat 1 tablespoon of oil in a large skillet on medium-high heat. Brown pork on one side until it is dark golden brown and releases from the pan, 3-5 minutes. Turn pieces and brown again on another side, repeating until pork is browned all over. Transfer meat to crock pot. Pour 1 ½ cups of water into skillet, turn heat to high, and scrape up all of the browned bits and pour into the crock pot. Add remaining tablespoon of garlic-infused oil, salt, pepper, vinegar, and brown sugar to slow cooker (do not add barbecue sauce yet). Cover and cook on low until pork can be shredded, 6-7 hours.
- Remove pork from slow cooker and shred meat into a large bowl; cover and set aside. Discard leek leaves. Pour liquid from the slow cooker into a large skillet. Bring to a boil and cook until reduced to 1 ½ cups, about 15 minutes. Pour liquid over meat and add 1 cup barbecue sauce, stirring to combine. Serve on low-FODMAP hamburger buns, passing additional barbecue sauce.

Serving: 12

together and rub them onto the pork: 1 teaspoon cumin, 1 teaspoon dry mustard, 1 teaspoon smoked paprika, 1 teaspoon ancho chile powder, 1 tablespoon packed brown sugar, ½ teaspoon salt, ¼ teaspoon black pepper.

Nutrition (per serving): 335 calories, 7.7g carbohydrates, 36.4g protein, 17.2g total fat, 278.1mg sodium, 1.3g fiber, 32.7mg calcium.

Barbecue Sauce

Commercial barbecue sauce contains onions, garlic and high-fructose corn syrup. When you make your own garlic- and onion-free sauce, you can adjust the sweetness to your taste, or add extra heat. The list of spices is long, but you will find that this tastes just like the real thing. The sauce freezes well so make a double batch.

¼ teaspoon asafetida (optional)
½ teaspoon salt
½ teaspoon ground black pepper
2 tablespoons dry mustard powder
1 teaspoon ground coriander
2 teaspoons ground cumin
1 tablespoon ancho chile powder
2 teaspoons smoked paprika
¼ teaspoon allspice
2 tablespoons Garlic- and Onion-Infused Oil
    (page 124)
½ cup finely minced leek leaves, green part only
1 ½ cups canned tomato puree or sauce (no garlic
    or onion added)
½ cup packed light brown sugar
⅓ cup white vinegar
1 tablespoon liquid smoke
2 cups water

Substitutions: Scallion greens can be used in place of leek greens. 2 tablespoons prepared mustard can be used in place of dry mustard. Any mild chile powder may be used in place of ancho. Mild or hot smoked paprika can be used, depending on heat preference. Granulated sugar may be used in place of brown sugar.

Nutrition (per serving): 41 calories, 5.9g carbohydrates, <1g protein, 2g total fat, 106mg sodium, <1g fiber, 18.7mg calcium.

- Combine spices, asafetida through allspice, in a small bowl and set aside.
- Heat the oil in a 2-quart saucepan on medium-high. Sauté leek leaves in the oil until soft, 2-3 minutes. Stir in dry spices for 1 minute. Add remaining ingredients and 2 cups of water. Bring to a boil, then reduce heat to a low simmer. Cook, stirring every few minutes and scraping pan sides and bottom with a rubber spatula, until sauce is slightly thinner than traditional barbecue sauce, about 30 minutes. Sauce will thicken as it cools. If it becomes too thick while simmering, add more water, ¼ cup at a time. Adjust with additional vinegar or brown sugar, to taste. Use within 5 days or freeze for extended storage.

Servings: 18, 2 tablespoons each. Yield: 2 ¼ cups

Ratatouille Casserole

This traditional dish from Provence is extra special when baked into a casserole with cheese.

Cheese filling:
1 large egg
2 cups lactose-free cottage cheese
½ teaspoon dried basil
½ teaspoon dried oregano
½ cup shredded Parmesan cheese (2 ounces)

Vegetables:
2 tablespoons garlic-infused oil, divided
1 unpeeled eggplant (1 ¼ pounds), cut into 1-inch cubes
1 red bell pepper, seeded and cut into ½-inch pieces
2 small yellow summer squash (1 pound), cut into ¼-inch rounds
2 small zucchini (1 pound), cut into ¼-inch rounds
1 ½ teaspoons dried basil
1 teaspoon dried oregano
½ teaspoon dried thyme
½ teaspoon salt
1 (14.5-ounce) can diced tomatoes (without added garlic or onion)
4 scallions, green part only, thinly sliced
Several generous grinds black pepper

Topping:
½ cup shredded Parmesan cheese (2 ounces)
¾ cup corn flake crumbs or Oven-Baked Breadcrumbs (page 130)

Tips: Cut recipe in half and bake in 9 x 9-inch baking pan

Variations: Omit the filling and topping. Instead, serve the ratatouille on pasta, polenta, or rice, sprinkled with Parmesan cheese.

Nutrition (per serving): 198 calories, 16.6g carbohydrates, 15.7g protein, 8.7g total fat, 583.4mg sodium, 5.4g fiber, 228.6mg calcium.

- Preheat oven to 400° F. Coat a 9 x 13-inch pan with baking spray or oil.
- In a medium bowl, beat egg with a fork. Stir in cottage cheese, herbs, and grated Parmesan cheese. Set aside.
- Heat 1 tablespoon of oil in a Dutch oven or large saucepan on medium-high heat. Sauté eggplant in the oil until it begins to brown, 2-3 minutes. Add red pepper and sauté until eggplant and peppers soften, 4-6 minutes. Transfer eggplant mixture to a large bowl and set aside.
- Add the remaining tablespoon of olive oil to the saucepan, along with summer squash, zucchini, herbs, and salt. Sauté until squash softens slightly, 2-3 minutes. Pour in canned tomatoes and their juices. Cook over medium heat and stir periodically until squash is soft but still slightly crunchy. Transfer vegetables to eggplant mixture in the bowl and add scallion greens and pepper. Spread half of the vegetables into the baking pan. Dollop cheese mixture evenly over vegetables and spread to cover. Spoon remaining vegetables over the cheese layer and bake until hot and bubbling, 30-35 minutes. Remove casserole from oven.
- Move oven rack to the top position and turn on broiler.
- Combine corn flake crumbs with Parmesan cheese and sprinkle evenly over the top of the ratatouille. Return casserole to the top rack of the oven and broil until topping is golden brown, 3-5 minutes.

Servings: 8

Savory Sausage and Kale Bread Pudding

This dish is a great way to introduce kale to your family. Kale pairs well with sausage, but ready-made sausage often contains garlic and onions. This recipe recreates the sausage taste without using high FODMAP ingredients.

12 ounces low-FODMAP bread
4 teaspoons garlic-infused oil
1 ½ cups seeded, chopped red or green bell
    pepper
7 cups thinly sliced kale leaves (¼ pound)
1 pound extra-lean ground pork
1 teaspoon fennel seeds, lightly chopped
1 teaspoon dried oregano
½ teaspoon smoked or regular paprika
½ teaspoon crushed red pepper flakes (optional)
¾ teaspoon salt
½ teaspoon ground black pepper
4 scallions, green part only, finely sliced
1 cup crumbled feta cheese (4 ounces)
5 large eggs
2 ½ cups lactose-free milk
1 teaspoon dry mustard powder or 1 tablespoon
    Dijon-style mustard

- Preheat oven to 350° F. Coat a 9 x 13-inch baking pan with baking spray or oil.
- Toast bread in a toaster until golden brown. Cut bread into 1-inch pieces and place in an extra-large mixing bowl.
- Heat the oil in a large skillet on medium-high heat. Sauté bell peppers in the oil until slightly soft, about 2 minutes. Add kale leaves and stir until wilted, 2-3 minutes. Scrape peppers and kale into mixing bowl with bread cubes. Sauté ground pork in the skillet over medium heat, breaking up the meat and stirring until meat is brown and crumbled. Stir in fennel, oregano, paprika, red pepper flakes, salt, and pepper. Add pork to the mixing bowl, along with scallion greens and feta cheese.
- In a medium bowl, beat eggs. Whisk in milk and mustard. Pour egg mixture over bread and vegetables, and stir to combine. Transfer the mixture to the prepared baking pan. Cover with foil and bake for 30 minutes. Remove foil and bake until top is golden brown, slightly puffy, and springs back when touched, approximately 20 more minutes.

Servings: 8

Tips: You can toast bread slices on a large baking tray in the oven for 8-10 minutes; turn slices over and bake until golden brown, 2-4 minutes more, instead of using a toaster. If you don't have a very large mixing bowl, you could use an 8-quart stock pot as a vessel. If you are unable to buy at least 90% lean pork, drain excess fat from browned meat before continuing with the recipe. To remove kale leaves from ribs: With one hand hold the stem end, with the other hand, pinch leaf halves firmly together where stem and leaf meet and quickly slide pinched fingers along rib toward the tip of the leaf. You will be left with a bare rib in one hand and two leaf halves in the other. Stack several leaves, roll up lengthwise, and slice roll crosswise.

Substitutions: Two drained, chopped, roasted bell peppers from a jar can be used instead of fresh red pepper; do not sauté. 6 ounces Swiss chard or fresh spinach can be used in place of kale.

Variations: Add 10-12 sliced, pitted black Kalamata olives

Time savers: Buy pre-washed, chopped kale or use a 10-ounce package of frozen spinach or kale (thaw and press out water).

Nutrition (per serving): 455 calories, 43.4g carbohydrates, 26.7g protein, 19.5g total fat, 583.9mg sodium, 3.1g fiber, 306.5mg calcium.

Steak with Chimichurri Sauce

This lively dish is from Argentina. Garlic oil is a must for the flavor of the sauce. You can buy commercial garlic oil or make your own (page 123). Though Chimichurri Sauce is traditionally served over steak, it also goes well with chicken, pork, fish, or shrimp. It can even be used as a vegetable or bread dip, or as a salad dressing. Plan ahead: the sauce is best prepared at least 1 hour and up to 1 day in advance to allow flavors to blend.

Chimichurri Sauce:
1 ½ cups flat leaf parsley, packed (about 1 bunch)
5 scallions, green part only, cut into 2-inch pieces
1 teaspoon ground cumin
1 ½ teaspoons smoked paprika
1 tablespoon dried oregano
¼ cup wine vinegar
½ teaspoon crushed red pepper flakes (optional)
½ teaspoon salt
¼ teaspoon ground black pepper
⅓ cup garlic-infused oil
Spice Rub:
1 teaspoon cumin
1 teaspoon smoked paprika
1 teaspoon coriander
½ teaspoon salt
½ teaspoon ground black pepper
2 tablespoons garlic-infused oil
2 pounds flank steak

- Measure parsley, scallion greens, cumin, smoked paprika, and oregano into a food processor and pulse several times until coarsely chopped. Add vinegar, 3 tablespoons water, red pepper flakes, salt, and pepper and pulse to combine. With the machine running, slowly pour in the oil. Process until the sauce is still slightly chunky. Do not puree smooth.
- Mix cumin, smoked paprika, coriander, salt, pepper, and oil in a small bowl. Brush mixture on both sides of the steak. Grill, broil, or pan fry steak until desired degree of doneness.
- To serve, top each cooked steak with two tablespoons of sauce. Serve extra sauce at the table.

Servings: 6

Tips: If using a blender, measure all Chimichurri ingredients into the bowl and blend until uniformly chunky. If you don't have a food processor or blender, finely chop herbs with a knife and whisk ingredients together in a small bowl.

Substitutions: Skirt, rib eye, strip, or sirloin steak can be used in place of flank steak. ¼ teaspoon cayenne pepper can be used instead of ½ teaspoon crushed red pepper flakes.

Variations: A mixture of 1 cup parsley and ½ cup cilantro leaves can be used for a flavor variation.

Time saver: Skip the spice rub; instead generously sprinkle the steak with salt and black pepper.

Nutrition (per serving): 395 calories, 3.2g carbohydrates, 34.9g protein, 27.11g total fat, 467.1mg sodium, 1.8g fiber, 75.5mg calcium.

Smoked paprika—a low-FODMAP staple

Smoked paprika, sometimes labeled Pimentón de la Vera, is a Spanish spice made from ground, smoked chile peppers and is a must for the pantry. It adds a nice smoky flavor to any dish. It comes in three heat levels: mild (dulce), moderate heat (agridulce), and hot (picante). Most supermarkets stock the mild variety. The recipes in this book call for the mild version, which is the most versatile. You can always add heat to recipes with cayenne pepper, crushed red pepper, or chile pepper.

What to do with all those scallion bulbs?
1. Serve them separately on the table for others to enjoy. While it is fine for people who don't have IBS to eat low-FODMAP food, in most cases the whole family should not be on a totally low-FODMAP diet. We recommend that most people continue to eat the fiber from all kinds of vegetables as part of a healthy diet.
2. Store them in the freezer until you have a few minutes to make Onion-Infused Oil (page 123)
3. Replant them in the garden—they will grow new greens. Store the cut ends in a bowl of water in the refrigerator until gardening day. Plant them so that the roots are just below the soil surface and the white part is poking out. Water them regularly and within a few weeks you will be able to harvest fresh scallion greens. You can regrow the scallions in a glass of water on the windowsill, too!

Turkey Meatloaf

One night, when Lisa was out of low-FODMAP breadcrumbs, she used oats and no one was the wiser that she was sneaking fiber into this family-friendly meal. Make a spare meatloaf to serve later: Double the recipe, bake both meatloaves and serve one immediately; cool the extra one and double wrap it for the freezer.

¾ cup uncooked rolled oats
½ cup lactose-free milk
3 tablespoons ground chia seeds
2 large eggs, lightly beaten
¼ cup of Lisa's Ketchup (page 126)
1 heaping teaspoon dried basil
1 heaping teaspoon dried oregano
¼ teaspoon ground black pepper
1 teaspoon salt
1 ½ pounds extra-lean ground turkey or ground
    beef
¼ cup sliced scallions, green part only

- Preheat oven to 350° F. Lightly coat a 9 x 5-inch loaf pan with baking spray or oil.
- Combine oats, chia seeds, and milk in a small bowl, and let sit until milk is absorbed, about 5 minutes.
- Beat eggs in a large mixing bowl. Mix in ketchup, basil, oregano, salt, pepper, and scallion greens. Stir in oat mixture. Using hands, break turkey or beef into golf-ball-sized pieces and add to the bowl. Gently mix the ingredients together until combined. Do not over-mix or texture will be tough. Bake until meatloaf reaches 160° F in the center, about 1 hour. Drain any fat that has accumulated in the baking pan before serving.

Servings: 8

Tips: For faster baking time, make individual portions in a muffin pan. Coat muffin cups with baking spray, fill each cup with meatloaf, and bake until 160° F in the center, about 25-30 minutes.

Variations: Add 5-6 ounces of spinach leaves, sautéed. Add ⅔ cup grated carrot. For a Mexican version, use 1 tablespoon Chili Powder Mix (page 125) in place of basil, oregano, and pepper.

Nutrition (per serving): 270 calories, 9.4g carbohydrates, 22.1g protein, 16.2g total fat, 448.7mg sodium, 2.1g fiber, 53.8mg calcium.

Stir-Fried Shrimp with Pineapple and Peanuts

This sweet and sour tropical stir-fry is infinitely adaptable to whatever vegetables you have on hand. Be sure to prepare all of the ingredients in advance as this goes together quickly once the cooking starts. Delicious served over warm rice or rice noodles.

Sauce:
3 ½ tablespoons reduced-sodium soy sauce or tamari
3 tablespoons rice wine vinegar
1 tablespoon cornstarch
¼ cup Lisa's Chicken Stock (page 146) or water
3 tablespoons packed light brown sugar
Stir-fry:
1 pound bok choy
1 red bell pepper, seeded and cut into thin strips
1 large carrot, peeled, cut on the bias (⅛-inch thick) to create ovals
2 teaspoons fresh ginger, peeled and finely minced
2 cups (about 12 ounces) fresh pineapple cut into ¼-inch pieces
3 scallions, green part only, thinly sliced
1 pound medium, peeled, raw shrimp
½ cup dry roasted peanuts
4 teaspoons canola or peanut oil, divided

Substitutions: Baby bok choy (no need to separate stems from leaves), Swiss chard, or fresh spinach can be used instead of full-sized bok choy. Cut crosswise into 1-inch thick pieces, rinse and drain. Chicken, cut into 1-inch pieces, can be used in place of shrimp. Canned, drained pineapple may be used in place of fresh pineapple.

Nutrition (per serving): 360 calories, 26.9g carbohydrates, 29.8g protein, 16.1g total fat, 194.7mg sodium, 6.2g fiber, 133mg calcium.

- Whisk together soy sauce, vinegar, cornstarch, chicken stock, and 3 tablespoons of water until the mixture is smooth. Whisk in brown sugar. Set aside.
- Cut about ½-inch from the root end of the bok choy and discard. Cut the white stalks from the leaves and slice them into 1-inch pieces. Slice leaves crosswise 1-inch thick. Rinse, drain, set aside, keeping leaves separate from stalks.
- Heat a wok or large skillet on high heat with 2 teaspoons of oil. Stir-fry shrimp in the oil until cooked through, 3-4 minutes. Transfer shrimp to a large bowl. Add 2 teaspoons of oil to the wok. Add red bell pepper and stir-fry for 1 minute, add carrots and stir-fry until brown spots appear, about 1 minute. Clear a space in the center of the wok or skillet and add ginger. Let sit for 30-45 seconds, and then mix in the vegetables from the sides. Add bok choy stalks and stir-fry until softer and more translucent, about 2 minutes. Add pineapple and bok choy leaves, stirring until leaves are wilted.
- Mix in scallion greens, shrimp, and stir-fry sauce. Bring sauce to a boil, stirring periodically, until sauce thickens and coats food, 1-2 minutes. Remove from heat, and top with peanuts. Serve with cooked rice or rice noodles.

Servings: 4

Side Dishes

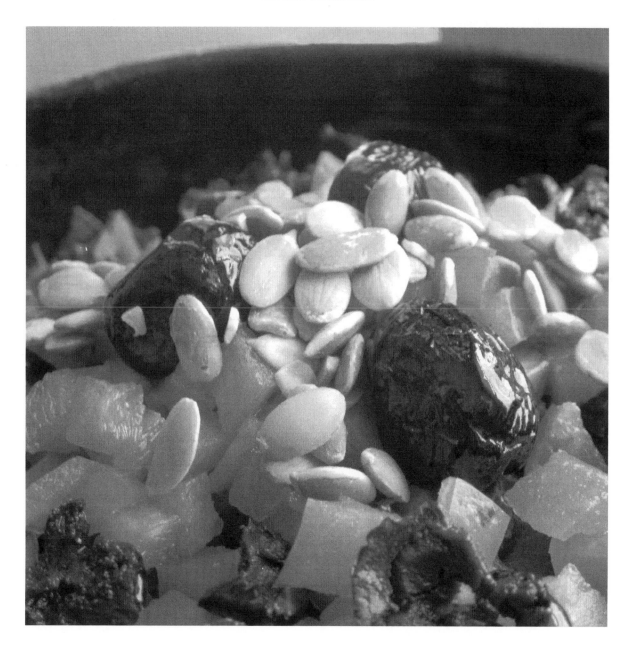

Smoky Kale Salad with Pumpkin Seeds and Shaved Parmesan

Kale's hardy texture and taste pair well with the bold flavors of smoked paprika, Parmesan, and oil-cured olives. Lisa's friends have said it is the best kale salad, ever! Allow time for this salad to marinate for at least 30 minutes before serving. Kale greens, particularly curly kale, are so hardy the salad can be prepared up to 8 hours in advance and leftovers are still tasty the next day. For a powerhouse salad, top with a cooked grain (quinoa, millet, sorghum, brown rice), grilled meat, or canned tuna.

¼ cup Lemon Vinaigrette (page 129)
¾ teaspoon smoked paprika
8 cups thinly sliced kale leaves, ribs removed (4 ounces)
8 black oil-cured olives, pitted and finely chopped
½ red bell pepper, seeded and diced into ¼-inch pieces
¼ cup shaved Parmesan cheese (1 ounce)
¼ cup pumpkin seeds (pepitas) or sunflower seeds

- Whisk vinaigrette and smoked paprika together in a large serving bowl. Add sliced kale, olives, and bell pepper and toss salad to coat with dressing. Hold at room temperature for 30 minutes, stirring every few minutes. Salad will wilt slightly. Top with pumpkin seeds just before serving.

Servings: 6

Tips: Use a vegetable peeler to shave Parmesan from a wedge of cheese. Alternatively, cheese can be grated coarsely. Pastene brand canned oil-cured olives are widely available.

Substitutions: Pitted kalamata olives can be used in place of oil-cured olives.

Time savers: Washed and cut kale leaves can be purchased in the produce section of the grocery store. These may need some additional chopping to reduce them to small ribbons, which helps them soak up the flavorful dressing.

Nutrition (per serving): 159 calories, 12.5g carbohydrates, 7.9g protein, 10.2g total fat, 193mg sodium, 2.7g fiber, 178mg calcium.

Barbecue-Roasted Potato Wedges

This is a delicious variation on oven-roasted potatoes.

1 medium russet potato (8 ounces), scrubbed clean, skin on
1 medium sweet potato (8 ounces), scrubbed clean, skin on
2 tablespoons Barbecue Spice Paste (page 125)

- Preheat oven to 425° F. Coat a large baking sheet with baking spray or oil.
- Cut potatoes lengthwise into ½-inch thick wedges. Brush cut sides with spice paste and place cut side down on baking sheet. Roast until golden brown, 15-20 minutes. Turn potatoes over and roast until browned, 15-20 minutes more.

Servings: 4

Variations: For grilled potatoes, microwave whole potatoes (pierce each once) until slightly soft but center is still hard when pierced with a sharp knife (2-4 minutes high power). Cut potatoes into wedges, brush with spice paste, and finish cooking on a grill until grill marks appear and potatoes are cooked through

Nutrition (per serving): 128 calories, 29.3g carbohydrates, 2.9g protein, <1g total fat, 189.9mg sodium, 4.2g fiber, 37.4mg calcium.

Asian Bean Sprout Salad

Sprouts should be boiled briefly, a cooking method known as blanching, due to the risk of food poisoning from consuming raw sprouts. These lightly cooked sprouts are popular in Asia.

Salad:
8 ounces fresh mung bean sprouts
4 cups water
1 teaspoon salt
2 scallions, green part only, sliced
¼ teaspoon red pepper flakes (optional)
Dressing:
1 teaspoon garlic oil
1 teaspoon sesame oil
1 tablespoon soy sauce
1 ½ teaspoons sugar
½ teaspoon peeled, finely grated ginger root

Nutrition (per serving): 21 calories, 2.9g carbohydrates, 1g protein, <1g total fat, 290.1mg sodium, <1g fiber, 7.6mg calcium.

- Bring water and salt to a rolling boil in a medium saucepan. Add sprouts and push down with a spoon to submerge. Boil for 30 seconds. Drain sprouts and plunge them into a bowl of cold water mixed with several ice cubes until cool. Drain, pat dry with a paper towel, and transfer to a serving bowl, along with scallion greens and optional red pepper flakes.
- Whisk dressing ingredients together in a small bowl until sugar is dissolved. Pour over the sprout mixture in the serving bowl. Allow flavors to blend for 15 minutes, stirring a few times. Serve as a side salad.

Servings: 6

Orange and Carrot Salad

Prepare this light, refreshing salad ahead of time; it tastes best after flavors blend for 30 minutes.

3 cups peeled, julienned carrots (about 4 large, ¾ pound)
1 ½ tablespoons garlic-infused oil
1 teaspoon ground coriander seed
¼ teaspoon ground cumin
⅓ cup fresh orange juice
½ teaspoon sugar
⅛ teaspoon salt
½ teaspoon orange zest
1 scallion, green part only, finely sliced
2 tablespoons finely minced cilantro or parsley leaves

Tips: To julienne carrots, turn the knife diagonally across the carrot at a 45 degree angle and cut into ⅛-inch thick ovals. Stack several ovals and cut lengthwise into ⅛-inch wide strips.

Time savers: Use prepared carrot matchsticks, available in the produce section of the grocery store.

Nutrition (per serving): 66 calories, 8.4g carbohydrates, <1g protein, 3.6g total fat, 94.4mg sodium, 2.1g fiber, 28.9mg calcium.

- Place julienned carrots in a medium serving bowl. Heat oil, coriander, and cumin in a small skillet on medium heat and stir until spices smell fragrant and darken slightly, 1-2 minutes. Pour hot oil over carrots and stir. Add orange juice, sugar, and salt to the skillet and reduce orange juice by half (about 3 tablespoons), 3-4 minutes. Pour juice over carrots. Stir in zest, scallion greens, and cilantro. Let flavors blend for 15-30 minutes, stirring several times.

Servings: 6

Microwave Polenta

A quick and tasty polenta can be made in the microwave with very little stirring and attention—just don't tell your Nonna. Use a microwave-safe bowl at least two times larger in volume than the ingredients. Cooking time varies due to differences in microwave power.

1 cup stone-ground cornmeal
1 teaspoon salt
3 ½ cups water or Lisa's Chicken Stock (page 146)
1 tablespoon garlic-infused oil, optional

- Combine cornmeal, salt, water, and oil in a 2-quart microwave safe bowl, and stir until smooth. Cover bowl with a microwave-safe plate and cook on high power for 5 minutes. Remove cover and stir. Cover, return to microwave, cook 5 more minutes, and stir again. Continue microwaving in 2 minute increments on high power, stirring each time, until polenta is soft and no longer gritty. Serve topped with Eggplant Puttanesca (page 91).

Servings: 5

Tips: This recipe works for all different grinds of cornmeal from fine to coarse; however, cooking time and liquid amounts will vary, so you may need to tweak the recipe.

Variations: For a cheesy version, add ¾ cup cheddar, Parmesan, or Romano at the end of cooking. Stir and microwave briefly until cheese is melted. For a creamy version, use half water, half lactose-free milk.

Nutrition calculated using water (per serving): 112 calories, 18.8g carbohydrates, 2g protein, 3.6g total fat, 478.7mg sodium, 1.8g fiber, 6.8mg calcium.

Oven-Baked Polenta Fries

These fries are delicious as is or dipped into Oven-Roasted Tomato Sauce (page 87) or Romesco Sauce (page 98). Oven baked or pan-fried polenta requires planning ahead to chill the polenta before slicing and frying.

1 recipe Microwave Polenta (above)
2 teaspoons oil

- Coat an 8 x 8-inch baking pan with baking spray or oil. Pour hot polenta into pan, and smooth the top. Refrigerate until firm, about 2 hours.
- Preheat oven to 450° F. Coat a large baking pan with baking spray or oil.
- Turn pan upside down on a cutting board and rap sharply to release polenta.
- Slice chilled polenta into ½ x ½ x 3-inch pieces. Place pieces on a baking sheet and coat lightly with baking spray or oil. Bake until pieces are golden on the bottom, 20-25 minutes. Turn fries over and bake until golden, about 20 more minutes.

Variations: Sprinkle with ½ teaspoon basil and ¼ teaspoon oregano before baking. For pan-fried polenta, chill and cut as for polenta fries. Fry in a skillet on medium-high heat in 1 tablespoon of butter or oil until golden brown, about 3 minutes per side.

Nutrition (per serving): 128 calories, 18.8g carbohydrates, 2g protein, 5.4g total fat, 478.7mg sodium, 1.8g fiber, 6.8mg calcium.

Chayote Sauté

Pronounced chah YO tay, this pale green, pear-shaped vegetable is related to squash with a taste and texture similar to cucumber and zucchini. It has many names: Mexican squash, choko, mirliton, and vegetable pear, to name a few. The skin and large, soft seed can be chopped along with the vegetable, making prep so easy, and it cooks in minutes. If that hasn't sold you on trying chayote, uncut chayote keeps for about two weeks in the refrigerator. Try it in stir fries, casseroles, or pasta dishes. It is available in Latin, Asian, and Caribbean markets and some grocery stores.

1 chayote (just under ½ pound)
½ red bell pepper, seeded and cut into ½-inch
    strips
2 teaspoons garlic-infused oil
½ teaspoon dried thyme
½ teaspoon dried oregano
¼ teaspoon salt
Several grinds black pepper
2 scallions, green part only, thinly sliced

- Rinse the chayote, cut a thin slice off one "cheek," and place it cut side down on a cutting board. Slice lengthwise into ¼-inch thick pear-shaped slabs. Stack two pieces together at a time and slice lengthwise into ¼-inch wide strips. Cut strips across to make shorter lengths if you prefer.
- Heat oil in a large skillet on medium-high heat. Sauté bell pepper briefly, then let it sit for 1 minute. Add chayote, thyme, oregano, salt, and pepper and continue stirring periodically until chayote is slightly translucent and softened, but still crisp, 3-5 minutes. Remove from heat and stir in scallion greens.

Servings: 4

Variations: For *Mexican* chayote, replace thyme and oregano with ½ teaspoon cumin and 1 teaspoon ancho chile powder (or 1 ½ teaspoons Chili Powder Mix, page 125). Sauté and when done, remove from heat and add 1 tablespoon lime juice, scallion greens, and 2 tablespoons pepitas (pumpkin seeds). For *Indian* chayote, replace thyme and oregano with 1 teaspoon curry powder or garam masala and ½ teaspoon finely chopped fresh, peeled ginger, stir in scallion greens. For *Italian* style, replace thyme with 1 teaspoon dried basil. Add 4-6 diced cherry or grape tomatoes when adding chayote. When done, stir in 2 tablespoons chopped black olives and scallion greens.

Nutrition (per serving): 40 calories, 4.1g carbohydrates, <1g protein, 2.6g total fat, 265.1mg sodium, 2.2g fiber, 18.7mg calcium.

Lime Cabbage Slaw

This light, refreshing slaw goes particularly well with Beef Fajitas (page 85)and Fish Tacos (page 89) but can also be eaten as a side with other meats, fish, or seafood. This recipe can be made several hours ahead.

Dressing:
2 ½ tablespoons fresh lime juice (1-2 limes)
1 tablespoon garlic-infused oil
¼ teaspoon salt
1 ¼ teaspoons sugar
Salad:
2 cups finely shredded green cabbage (⅓ pound)
2 scallions, green part only, thinly sliced
3 tablespoons minced cilantro leaves

- Whisk dressing ingredients together in a large serving bowl. Stir in cabbage, scallion greens, and cilantro until vegetables are thoroughly coated with dressing. Allow flavors to blend for at least 15 minutes, stirring every few minutes.

Servings: 4

Variations: Add 1 teaspoon of Chili Powder Mix (page 125) or ½ teaspoon ancho chile powder plus ¼ teaspoon cumin. Add 1 carrot, grated or julienned.

Time savers: Buy prepared shredded cabbage in the produce section of the grocery store.

Nutrition (per serving): 50 calories, 4.9g carbohydrates, <1g protein, 3.5g total fat, 155.8mg sodium, 1.5g fiber, 25.4mg calcium.

Asian Rutabaga Coleslaw

Rutabaga may have originated as a cross between a cabbage and turnip and has a mild, sweet flavor when raw. It resembles a very large turnip (often 5 inches or more in diameter) and is sometimes labeled yellow turnip. The yellow and tan-purple skin is often coated in wax.

Coleslaw:
1 pound rutabaga, peeled and julienned
1 ½ cups peeled carrots, shredded (4 carrots, ¾ pound)
½ red bell pepper, seeded and thinly sliced into ½-inch long pieces
3 scallions, green part only, thinly sliced
Dressing:
2 tablespoons granulated sugar
5 tablespoons unseasoned rice vinegar
2 tablespoons toasted sesame oil
1 tablespoon canola oil
3 tablespoons reduced-sodium soy sauce
1 teaspoon peeled, minced ginger root
3 tablespoons sesame seeds

- Combine rutabaga, carrots, red bell pepper, and scallion greens in a serving bowl. Whisk together sugar, vinegar, sesame oil, canola oil, soy sauce, and ginger until sugar is dissolved. Pour dressing over coleslaw and toss to coat. Chill for 30 minutes, stirring several times. Sprinkle with sesame seeds before serving.

Servings: 8

Tips: If you have a food processor, you can grate the rutabaga instead.

Substitutions: 4 tablespoons minced chives can be used in place of scallion greens. ⅓ cup roasted peanuts may be used in place of sesame seeds.

Variations: Add one of the following: 2 red radishes, thinly sliced, 1 ½ cups blanched mung bean sprouts (see tips, page 82), or a 5-ounce can of water chestnuts, rinsed, drained, and coarsely chopped.

Time savers: Buy 12 ounces of prepared carrot matchsticks to use in place of grated carrots.

Nutrition (per serving): 125 calories, 18.1g carbohydrates, 2.2g protein, 7.1g total fat, 398.5mg sodium, 1.9g fiber, 82.1mg calcium.

Curried Quinoa Salad with Almonds

This cold salad is a great initiation dish for those who are afraid to try quinoa. Whenever Lisa brings this dish to a potluck it is always a hit.

Salad:
1 cup uncooked quinoa, rinsed
1 ¾ cup water
½ teaspoon salt, divided
3 scallions, green part only, finely sliced
1 cup red grapes, halved
½ cup sliced, toasted almonds
6 ounces baby spinach (optional for serving)
Dressing:
2 tablespoons extra virgin olive oil
½ teaspoon peeled, finely minced ginger
1 tablespoon mild curry powder
½ teaspoon ground coriander
1 teaspoon cumin
2 tablespoons fresh lime juice
2 teaspoons sugar

- Combine quinoa, 1¾ cups water, and ¼ teaspoon salt in a 2-quart saucepan on medium-high heat. Cover and bring to a boil. Reduce heat to a simmer and cook until you see the small yellow tail coming out of the grain, 12-13 minutes. Remove from heat, and let sit

Substitutions: Vinegar can be used in place of lime juice. Red quinoa can be substituted for the more common yellow/light brown quinoa; use 2 cups of water and simmer for slightly longer, 15-16 minutes.

Variations: Add sliced grilled chicken or grilled shrimp to the quinoa salad before serving; rub the chicken or grilled shrimp with Barbecue Spice Paste (page 125) before grilling for extra flavor.

Nutrition (per serving): 254 calories, 29.7g carbohydrates, 7.7g protein, 12.9g total fat, 211.2mg sodium, 4.7g fiber, 83.9mg calcium.

covered for 5 minutes. If there is any water remaining, drain it off and place cooked quinoa in a serving bowl.

- While quinoa is cooking, make the dressing. Add oil and ginger to a small skillet on medium heat. Stir until ginger sizzles, about 1 minute. Add curry powder, coriander, cumin, and remaining ¼ teaspoon of salt and heat on medium, stirring constantly until spices are fragrant and darken a shade, 1-2 minutes. Remove pan from the heat and stir in lime juice and sugar. Pour warm dressing over quinoa and stir. Mix in scallion greens and red grapes and chill mixture for at least 30 minutes. Top with nuts just before serving. Serve on a bed of baby spinach if desired.

Servings: 6

Fall Vegetable Sauté with Spicy Maple Glaze

This colorful skillet sauté is faster than roasting and still brings out the vegetables' natural sweetness and flavor. Any combination of low-FODMAP root vegetables works. Rutabaga (a.k.a. yellow waxed turnip) when lightly cooked is a surprisingly sweet and crunchy vegetable.

> 1 ½ cups peeled and sliced carrots (6 ounces, 2-3 medium)
> 1 ½ cups peeled and sliced parsnips (6 ounces, 2-3 medium)
> 1 ½ cups peeled and sliced rutabaga (6 ounces)
> 1 ½ cups peeled and sliced butternut squash (6 ounces)
> 1 ½ tablespoons butter
> 1 ½ teaspoons mild curry powder (optional)
> ½ teaspoon ground coriander (optional)
> ¼ cup water
> 3 tablespoons 100% pure maple syrup

- Peel and slice vegetables to make a total of 6 cups. Cutting all vegetable into uniform ¼-inch slices ensures even cooking.
- Melt butter on medium-high in a large skillet, sauté pan, or wok. Add curry powder and coriander to the pan and let it sit for 30 seconds. Stir in vegetables, letting them rest, and then stirring occasionally until they begin to brown, 4-5 minutes. Pour in ¼ cup water and stir. Cook until the vegetables are beginning to soften but are still slightly crunchy, 3-4 minutes. If vegetables are still too hard, add a tablespoon or two of water and sauté another minute. Add maple syrup and continue to stir until syrup caramelizes, about 1 minute.

Servings: 8

Tips: For parsnips and carrots, cut peeled carrots and parsnips into 2-inch lengths; cut pieces lengthwise in half; turn pieces flat side down, and cut each lengthwise into ¼-inch thick wedges. For butternut squash, peel skin from the neck of the butternut squash and cut crosswise into ¼-inch thick rounds; cut rounds into ¼-inch sticks. For rutabaga, cut a thin slice off the root end of rutabaga; place cut side down on surface and cut ¼-inch thick rounds; peel skin off edges of rounds; cut rounds into ¼-inch sticks; cut crosswise to make shorter 2-inch lengths.

Nutrition (per serving): 79 calories, 14.7g carbohydrates, <1g protein, 2.4g total fat, 22.3mg sodium, 2.7g fiber, 40.2mg calcium.

Middle Eastern Chopped Salad

Za'atar is a spice blend of sumac, a burgundy-colored spice with a tart, fruity taste, thyme, sesame seeds, and sometimes oregano or marjoram. Found in Middle Eastern markets or online, this versatile spice mix is worth seeking out. Homemade croutons replace the toasted pita that is typically added to the salad.

Salad:
½ **English cucumber, unpeeled, diced into ¼-inch pieces**
½ **red bell pepper, seeded and diced into ¼-inch pieces**
1 **large tomato, diced into ¼-inch pieces**
3 **scallions, green part only, thinly sliced**
½ **cup chopped parsley leaves**
6 **Kalamata olives, pitted, coarsely chopped**
4 **cups chopped romaine leaves**
¾ **cup Herbed Croutons (below)**

Dressing:
2 **tablespoons fresh lemon juice**
1 **tablespoon red wine vinegar**
2 **tablespoons garlic-infused oil**
¼ **teaspoon salt**
¼ **teaspoon pepper**
½ **teaspoon sugar**
2 **teaspoons za'atar**

- Combine cucumbers, red pepper, tomatoes, scallion greens, parsley, olives, lettuce, and croutons in a large serving bowl.
- Whisk together the dressing ingredients in a small bowl. Pour dressing over salad and toss to coat. Let sit 10 minutes, stirring several times to allow flavors to blend.

Servings: 6 side salads

Tips: The croutons will soak up the dressing and juices. If you prefer crunchier croutons, add just before serving salad.

Substitutions: One regular peeled cucumber may be used in place of the English cucumber.

Variations: For a dinner salad, add feta cheese and grilled chicken strips.

Nutrition (per serving): 88 calories, 7.8g carbohydrates, 1.5g protein, 6g total fat, 190.5mg sodium, 1.8g fiber, 34.1mg calcium.

Herbed Croutons

The recipe makes more croutons than you need for the salad. Leftovers, stored in an airtight container to keep them crisp and dry, will keep for several weeks.

3 **tablespoons garlic-infused oil**
1 **teaspoon dried basil**
½ **teaspoon dried oregano**
Scant ¼ **teaspoon salt**
Few grinds black pepper
8 **slices low-FODMAP bread**

- Preheat oven to 350° F.
- Combine oil, basil, oregano, salt, and pepper in a small bowl. Brush both sides of bread with mixture. Stack 2-3 bread slices and cut bread into ½-inch cubes. Repeat with remaining bread. Place bread cubes on a baking pan and bake until cubes are golden brown on the bottom, 8-10 minutes. Turn croutons over, turn oven down to 325° F. Bake until golden brown and crisp all over, 5-7 minutes. Let cool. If croutons have any soft spots, return pan to the oven, turn heat off, and leave the door slightly ajar for 10-15 minutes more.

Servings: 24 **Yield:** 3 cups

Nutrition (per serving): 31 calories, 3g carbohydrates, <1g protein, 1.9g total fat, 32.6mg sodium, <1g fiber, 6.6mg calcium.

Pan-Seared Cabbage

Searing brings out the sweet taste of the cabbage, which pairs well with the salty, smoky bacon.

½ head green cabbage (half of a 2 ½ pound
  cabbage)
2 pieces bacon
¼ teaspoon dried thyme or sage
⅛ teaspoon salt
Several grinds of black pepper
3 tablespoons balsamic vinegar
2 teaspoons granulated sugar

- Cut the half cabbage into 6 wedges through core, leaving core to hold each wedge together. Sprinkle wedges on cut sides with salt and pepper.
- Heat a large skillet on medium-high and cook bacon until crisp. Remove bacon and set aside, leaving bacon fat in the skillet. Place cabbage wedges in skillet cut side down and sear pieces without moving until very dark brown, 3-4 minutes. Turn wedges over, sprinkle with thyme, cover skillet and cook 3 minutes. Remove cover and add vinegar, sugar, and 2 tablespoons water to skillet. When the mixture bubbles, spoon juices over cabbage wedges. Boil until sauce thickens and coats the pan. Turn off heat and use a spatula to gently remove cabbage wedges onto a plate. Pour sauce over cabbage. Crumble bacon into small pieces and sprinkle over cabbage wedges.

Servings: 6

Variations: Omit bacon and use 1 tablespoon garlic-infused oil to sear cabbage, then add ½ teaspoon mild, smoked paprika when adding thyme.

Nutrition (per serving): 90 calories, 7.4g carbohydrates, 2.5g protein, 5.8g total fat, 169.5mg sodium, 2g fiber, 36mg calcium.

Sweet and Tangy Sautéed Radishes

Radishes are an oft-overlooked vegetable, probably due to their raw, peppery bite. Cooking eliminates the pungency, turning them into a tasty, approachable vegetable. We urge you to revisit the lowly radish since they are easy to find, and they add a bright color to dishes.

1 pound red radishes, trimmed (halve the largest
  radishes)
1 tablespoon butter
½ teaspoon dried thyme
¼ teaspoon salt
Several grinds black pepper
⅓ cup water
1 tablespoon granulated sugar
1 tablespoon vinegar

- Melt butter on medium-high in a 10-inch skillet. Sauté radishes, thyme, salt, and pepper in the butter for 1 minute, shaking pan several times. Add water and sugar, cover pan and bring to a boil. Reduce heat to low and cook for 3 minutes, shaking pan several times. Add vinegar and boil uncovered until the sauce is reduced to 2 tablespoons of syrupy glaze. Radishes are done when tender on the outside but still firm in the middle (test with a sharp knife). If radishes are done, but glaze is still thin, remove radishes from the pan and reduce sauce until syrupy. Pour the glaze over the cooked radishes and serve warm.

Servings: 4

Substitutions: Dried oregano or sage can be used in place of thyme.

Variations: Add 2 tablespoons minced chives or green part of scallion when cooking is done.

Nutrition (per serving): 57 calories, 7.4g carbohydrates, <1g protein, 3g total fat, 190.7mg sodium, 1.9g fiber, 32.2mg calcium.

Oven-Roasted Radishes

We roast other root vegetables; why not radishes?

1 pound red radishes, trimmed (halve the largest radishes)
1 tablespoon extra-virgin olive oil
¼ teaspoon dried thyme
¼ teaspoon dried sage
⅛ teaspoon salt
Several grinds black pepper

- Preheat oven to 450° F.
- Scatter radishes in a roasting pan, drizzle with olive oil and sprinkle with herbs, salt, and pepper. Roast until soft on the outside, yet a knife inserted in the middle encounters some resistance, about 18-20 minutes, shaking pan midway through roasting.

Servings: 4

Nutrition (per serving): 49 calories, 4.1g carbohydrates, <1g protein, 3.5g total fat, 117.1mg sodium, 1.9g fiber, 31.7mg calcium.

Roasted Fall Vegetable Salad with Maple Balsamic Vinaigrette

Roasted root vegetables become sweet, almost like candy. Kabocha squash does not need to be peeled, as the skin will soften, but you can peel it if you prefer. Use Grade B maple syrup for cooking and baking if you can find it, as it has a more pronounced maple flavor.

Roasted Vegetables:
2 cups kabocha squash, cut into 1-inch pieces
2 cups peeled rutabaga, cut into 1-inch pieces
2 teaspoons oil, plus extra for pan
½ teaspoon dried thyme
½ teaspoon dried sage leaves, crumbled
½ teaspoon salt
Several generous grinds black pepper
Maple Balsamic Vinaigrette:
⅓ cup balsamic vinegar
¼ cup walnut oil or canola oil
¼ cup 100% pure maple syrup
2 teaspoons Dijon mustard, or 1 teaspoon dry mustard
1 tablespoon reduced sodium soy sauce or tamari
Several grinds of black pepper
Salad:
12 cups mixed salad greens (12 ounces)
½ cup coarsely chopped toasted walnuts

- Preheat oven to 425° F. Lightly coat a baking sheet with oil.
- Toss vegetables with 2 teaspoons of oil, herbs, salt, and pepper. Roast on baking sheet until vegetables begin to brown, about 20 minutes. Turn pieces and cook 10-15 more minutes, until brown on the other side.
- Combine dressing ingredients in a tightly sealed container and shake until well blended. Warm the vinaigrette briefly in a microwave just before dressing the salad. Do not boil.
- Divide salad greens onto 6 plates. Top with the roasted vegetables, walnuts, and dressing.

Servings: 8

Tips: Kabocha squash is easier to cut if you first pierce the squash several times with a sharp knife and microwave it on high power for 3-4 minutes.

Substitutions: Other types of vinegar may be used in the dressing in place of balsamic. Carrots and parsnips can be used instead of kabocha and rutabaga.

Variations: Candied Maple-Spiced Nuts (page 134) can be used in place of walnuts. Add crumbled feta or goat cheese to the salad.

Time savers: Pre-washed greens can be purchased in the produce section of your grocery store.

Nutrition (per serving): 191 calories, 17.7g carbohydrates, 2.8g protein, 13g total fat, 254.8mg sodium, 3.3g fiber, 66.7mg calcium.

Rice Pilaf

Commercial rice pilaf mixes usually contain dried garlic and onion. When plain rice feels "ho hum," try this low-FODMAP version made flavorful by sautéing aromatic vegetables. See variations for several delicious flavor combinations.

1 tablespoon garlic-or garlic-onion-infused oil
¼ cup finely minced carrots
¼ cup finely minced peeled rutabaga
¼ cup finely minced, peeled celery root/celeriac
1 cup long grain white rice
2 cups Lisa's Chicken Stock (page 146) or water
⅓ cup sliced scallions, green part only
½ teaspoon turmeric
1 bay leaf
¼ teaspoon salt (if using water increase to ½
    teaspoon)
⅛ teaspoon ground black pepper
⅛ teaspoon asafetida
Herbs and spices of choice, see Variations
⅓ cup chopped toasted almonds, walnuts, pecans,
    or whole pine nuts (optional)

- Heat the oil in a 2-quart saucepan on medium-high heat. Add carrots, rutabaga, and celery root and stir periodically until golden brown, 3-4 minutes. Add rice and stir 1 ½ minutes. Add stock, half of the scallion greens, turmeric, bay leaf, salt, pepper, and herbs or spices of preference, see Variations. Cover and bring to a boil. Turn heat down to a low simmer. Cook for 18 minutes.
- Remove from heat. Let pilaf sit for 5-7 minutes. Uncover, fluff rice and stir in remaining scallion greens. Top with nuts and serve.

Servings: 6

Substitutions: Chopped kabocha squash, acorn squash, or sweet potato can be used in place of carrots.

Variations: For *herbed pilaf*, cook rice with ¼ teaspoon thyme, ¼ teaspoon oregano, ¼ teaspoon basil, garnish with ¼ cup chopped parsley. For *saffron pilaf*, omit turmeric and add ⅛ teaspoon crushed saffron threads. For *Indian pilaf*, omit turmeric and add 1 ½ teaspoons curry powder. For *Mexican pilaf*, omit carrots and turmeric and add ½ cup diced red bell pepper; add 1 tablespoon Chili Powder Mix (page 125) or 1 teaspoon cumin and 2 teaspoons ancho chile powder, garnish with ¼ cup minced cilantro leaves.

Nutrition (per serving): 201 calories, 28.6g carbohydrates, 5.9g protein, 7g total fat, 388.2mg sodium, 1.7g fiber, 47.3mg calcium.

Shaved Squash Salad with Mint and Feta

This refreshing salad tastes great as a side dish, or served over pasta.

¼ cup garlic-infused oil
2 tablespoons fresh lemon juice
½ teaspoon lemon zest
½ teaspoon salt
½ teaspoon ground black pepper
2 small yellow summer squash (about 1 pound,
    total)
2 small zucchini (about 1 pound, total)
3 tablespoons minced chives
⅓ cup coarsely chopped mint
¼ cup toasted, chopped walnuts or almonds
¼ cup crumbled feta cheese (1 ounce)

- Whisk olive oil, lemon juice, zest, salt, and black pepper together in a small bowl.
- Shave summer squash and zucchini lengthwise into long strips using a Spiralizer or vegetable peeler. Place in a large serving bowl and add dressing. Mix in chives, mint, walnuts, and feta cheese. Allow salad to marinate for 20 minutes before serving, stirring gently several times.

Servings: 6

Substitutions: Shaved Parmesan cheese can be used instead of feta cheese (shave with vegetable peeler).

Nutrition (per serving): 155 calories, 6.8g carbohydrates, 3.6g protein, 13.8g total fat, 279.6mg sodium, 2.2g fiber, 64.7mg calcium.

Simple Bell Pepper Sauté

Sautéed bell peppers can be served over burgers, in tacos, with eggs, or as a side dish with almost anything.

1 ½ teaspoons garlic-infused oil
2 red bell peppers, seeded and cut into ¼-inch
    strips
¼ teaspoon dried thyme
⅛ teaspoon salt
Few grinds black pepper
2 tablespoons balsamic vinegar
½ teaspoon sugar

Variations: Use a combination of red, yellow, orange, and green peppers for a colorful dish.

Nutrition (per serving): 47 calories, 6.5g carbohydrates, <1g protein, 1.9g total fat, 77.6mg sodium, 1.6g fiber, 9.8mg calcium.

- Heat the oil in a large skillet on medium-high. Add peppers, sauté for 3-5 minutes until pieces turn brown in spots, with some specks of black. Add thyme, salt, pepper, and 3 tablespoons of water. Cover pan with a lid until peppers are soft but still have some crunch, 2-4 minutes. Remove cover, let water boil off. Stir in vinegar and sugar. Vinegar will thicken, reduce, and coat the peppers. Serve warm or cold.

Servings: 4

Smashed Potatoes

These are Lisa's family's new favorite potato, replacing French fries as a treat.

1 ½ pounds red-skinned potatoes, each about 2-
    inch in diameter, washed, skin on
3 tablespoons garlic-infused oil
1 teaspoon crushed, dried rosemary
½ teaspoon dried thyme
½ teaspoon salt, divided
Several generous grinds black pepper

Tips: Potatoes can be made in advance and reheated at 300° F for 15-20 minutes. Potatoes can be finished on the grill. Precook as above, brush both sides with oil, and grill on each side with the grill cover down until potatoes turn light golden with grill marks.

Nutrition (per serving): 225 calories, 30.9g carbohydrates, 3.6g protein, 10.3g total fat, 301.3mg sodium, 2.9g fiber, 16.9mg calcium.

- Preheat oven to 425° F. Coat a baking sheet with 1 tablespoon of oil.
- Place potatoes on a microwave safe plate. Microwave potatoes until soft, but just slightly undercooked. A sharp knife inserted into the potato should go in with slight resistance at the center. Put potato on a smooth surface. Place the bottom of a plate or saucepan on top of potato and gently apply pressure to flatten the potato to ⅓- ½-inch thick round. The potato should stay together, but if a few small pieces break off press them back into the round. If potatoes are hard and crumbling when pressed, they are not cooked enough. Microwave longer until soft enough to flatten.
- Gently transfer smashed potatoes with a spatula to the baking sheet in a single layer with space in between each one. Brush potatoes with oil, sprinkle with ¼ teaspoon salt, chopped rosemary, thyme, and pepper. Bake until potatoes have formed a golden brown crust on the bottom, 20-25 minutes. Gently turn potatoes over, sprinkle with remaining salt and bake until golden, about 20 minutes more. Serve hot.

Servings: 4

Thanksgiving Wild Rice and Sausage Stuffing

Year after year Lisa tried to make stuffing from wheat-free bread cubes, but it always turned out mushy. Ditching that idea, she came up with this stuffing as a tasty replacement that has become a family favorite. This recipe can be made a day ahead and reheated in a microwave, freeing up premium oven space on Thanksgiving Day. This is a great side dish any time of the year. Stuffing leftovers can be quickly turned into a soup.

4 cups Lisa's Chicken Stock (page 146) or water
2 ½ cups water
1 ¼ cups uncooked wild rice
2 bay leaves
1 ¼ teaspoons salt, divided
1 ¼ cups uncooked long grain brown rice
1 pound extra-lean ground pork
1 fennel bulb, stalks and core removed, diced into
    ¼-inch pieces
¼ cup diced celery root/celeriac
1 large parsnip (6 ounces), peeled, diced into ¼-
    inch pieces
3 tablespoons finely minced fresh sage leaves
1 ¼ teaspoons dried thyme
6 scallions, green part only, thinly sliced
½ teaspoon ground black pepper
¾ cup of lightly chopped, toasted pecans
    (optional)

Tips: Leftovers make a hearty soup. Add some chopped carrots, rutabaga, and bell pepper to Lisa's Chicken Stock (page 146) and simmer until soft. Add rice stuffing, stirring until hot. How easy is that?

Substitutions: 1 tablespoon dried sage leaves or 1 teaspoon dry, rubbed sage can be used in place of fresh sage.

Nutrition (per serving): 212 calories, 25.9g carbohydrates, 9.2g protein, 9g total fat, 218.4mg sodium, 3.2g fiber, 31mg calcium.

- Combine 4 cups chicken stock, 2 ½ cups of water, wild rice, bay leaves, and 1 teaspoon salt in a Dutch oven or large stockpot; cover and bring to a boil. Turn heat down to simmer and cook for 10 minutes. Stir in brown rice, cover, and simmer until rice is tender but not mushy, about 40 minutes. Remove pot from the heat and let sit covered for 15 minutes. Drain any liquid that isn't absorbed and discard bay leaves.
- While rice is cooking, sauté pork in a large skillet on medium-high heat until golden brown and crumbled. Spoon cooked pork into a large mixing bowl, leaving 2 tablespoons of pork drippings in the pan. Add fennel, celery root, parsnip, sage, thyme, and remaining ¼ teaspoon salt to the pan and sauté on medium-high until vegetables are soft and lightly browned, 10-12 minutes. Combine sautéed vegetables with the pork. Stir in scallion greens, cooked rice, and pepper. Adjust taste with additional salt, pepper, and herbs, if needed. Stuffing can be served right away or placed in a greased 3-quart casserole to be reheated later. Top with chopped pecans just before serving.

Servings: 15, ¾ cups each.

Fresh or dried herbs?

If you are fortunate enough to have an herb garden or your budget permits you to buy fresh herbs year-round, they can be used in savory recipes instead of dried herbs. Use a 1:3 rule of thumb:

1 teaspoon dried herbs = 3 teaspoons of fresh herbs

Sauces and Seasonings

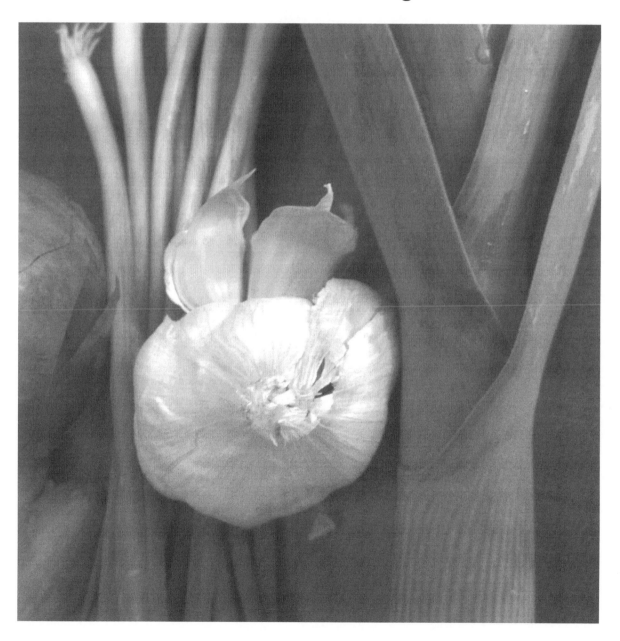

The No-Onion, No-Garlic Challenge

Garlic, onions, leeks, shallots, green onions (also known as spring onions or scallions), and ramps are all part of the allium family and are problematic for most people with IBS. Since garlic and onions are the cornerstone of flavor building in almost every cuisine, these are the most difficult FODMAPs to avoid. In addition, many ready-made spice mixes (chili powder, seasoned salt, taco seasoning, spice rubs, etc.) that we use routinely to flavor our foods contain garlic and/or onion powder, which are also off limits. Cooking without these flavorings often leaves dishes tasting flat and one-dimensional. There are ways around this cooking conundrum, and these techniques will soon become an easy part of your new food preparation style. This chapter also provides recipes for many tasty spice mixes that you can make yourself without garlic or onion powder, so you won't have to live without flavorful foods.

The best technique for adding onion flavor to foods is to use the green parts of scallions, chives, and leek leaves (yes, the portion you usually throw away). The green parts of these plants are much lower in FODMAPs than the white portion and are usually well tolerated. To add a burst of onion flavor, use the green part of scallions and chives near the end, or just after the dish finishes cooking. Alternatively, add about ⅔ of the green portions of scallions and chives at the beginning of cooking and save the remaining ⅓ to add to the dish when done cooking. When making broths, soups, stews, or sauces that cook longer, add the green part of scallions, chives, or leek leaves in the beginning to infuse the dish with onion flavor. Since leek leaves are quite tough, they need at least 10-15 minutes of cooking to soften, so always add them early on in cooking. Because of this, Lisa prefers leek leaves as the flavoring agent for soups and stews which simmer for long periods of time. Ask your friends who cook to save the green part of leeks for you. They freeze well, especially when sliced. This can also be done with the green part of scallions and chives. They will all darken and soften upon thawing and won't look bright green, but will still taste oniony.

Chives, which are used often in this book, and their cousin, garlic chives, grow in fast-spreading clumps in full sun or partial shade. At the end of summer, these plants can be harvested, minced, and frozen to use throughout the winter. You can also divide the clumps, to increase your crop or share with others. In two years, Lisa's first chive plant has grown to 10 large plants producing about 4 cups of minced chives to freeze!

It is possible to extract some of the flavor components of garlic and onions into oil to make garlic- or onion-infused oil, as the oil-soluble fractions of garlic and onions are low in FODMAPs. There are three options for garlic- or onion-infused oil:

1. Commercially prepared garlic-infused oil for cooking is available. Avoid products containing garlic extract (juice). This is a good solution for a short-term elimination diet; however, it can become expensive if you need to limit onions and garlic long-term. Commercially prepared garlic- or onion-infused oils are safe for extended storage because the FDA requires commercial preparations of garlic-, herb-, and onion-infused oils to be acidified, which prevents the growth of botulism spores. This technique is not available to the home cook.

2. To infuse a single dish with garlic and/or onion, heat the oil of your choice in a pan. Add coarsely chopped garlic cloves and/or onions. Sauté gently on medium heat for a few minutes, and then remove the garlic and onion pieces from the oil with a slotted spoon. To avoid bitterness, do not allow the garlic or onion to brown.

3. Make your own garlic- and/or onion-infused oil. This is economical and tasty, but there is risk of serious botulism poisoning if these homemade oils are not stored correctly. Numerous botulism poisonings have resulted from people ingesting garlic-infused oil, herb-infused oils, and vegetables marinated in oil (ex: roasted peppers, mushrooms, eggplant). All soil contains the bacteria Clostridium botulinum, therefore any soil-grown plant stored in oil can introduce Clostridium botulinum spores into the oil. These bacteria produce botulism toxin at room temperature in a low acid, oxygen-free environment, which are the exact conditions that oil provides. **You cannot taste, smell or see botulism toxin or spores in the oil. Furthermore, boiling and heating will not kill the spores!** Please read the following safe storage information carefully before making your own garlic-infused oil:

Never store any homemade garlic-, onion-, or herb-infused oils at room temperature. Label the oil with the date and store in the refrigerator for no more than 4 days. Discard oil if it has been left out of the refrigerator. Some oils may turn cloudy when refrigerated, but this does not affect the taste, is not an indicator of spoilage, and the oil will clear when warmed up.

For long-term storage, freezing the oil is safe as the botulism bacteria cannot grow at these low temperatures. Freezer storage is indefinite if the oil remains frozen; however, time may affect the taste and quality of the oil. The oil will solidify in the freezer, but will be soft enough to scrape portions out (a fork or serrated spoon are best). If you suspect the oil has thawed or been left out at room temperature, discard it. For quick thawing, remove only the amount of oil that is needed for the recipe and keep the remainder frozen. A few minutes at room temperature or a second or two in a hot pan or microwave will thaw it immediately.

Any dish made with homemade infused oils, such as salad dressing, should be refrigerated and consumed within 4 days, or frozen for longer term storage.

Another way to add onion and garlic flavor is to use a spice called asafetida powder (a.k.a. hing), found in Indian markets. It contains neither garlic nor onion, but it has a strong, distinctive smell and taste of onion and garlic. Use ⅛-¼ teaspoon in a small recipe, or ½-¾ teaspoon in a large stew or soup. Don't be put off by the strong smell, as it will disappear when cooked. Those with celiac disease should look for a certified gluten-free product, as some asafetida powders contain wheat flour. Such small amounts of wheat are not usually problematic for those with IBS.

Eventually, some people with IBS find that they can tolerate some small amounts of onions and garlic. When you are feeling better, you may want to try to figure out your personal tolerance level. This will vary from person to person. Hopefully you will find you can tolerate eating them on an occasional basis, such as when you are eating out at a restaurant or a friend's home. You might even be able to use small amounts regularly in your own cooking.

Garlic-Infused Oil

Increase or decrease the amount of garlic to your preference.

½ cup extra-virgin oil
8-10 peeled, coarsely chopped garlic cloves

- Heat oil and chopped garlic in a very small skillet on medium-high so that the garlic is immersed in the oil. When oil bubbles, turn heat to low to maintain a slow bubble. Simmer just until garlic turns pale yellow, about 4 minutes. Do not brown or it will be bitter. Remove from heat and let sit a few minutes. Pour oil through a fine sieve or cheesecloth. Refrigerate garlic-infused oil immediately and discard after 4 days, or freeze for long-term storage.

Yield: ⅓ cup

Tip: Store infused oil in glass or ceramic containers because plastic can crack when scooping out frozen oil.

Substitutions: Any type of oil can be used in place of olive oil.

Nutrition (entire recipe): 630 calories, 0g carbohydrates, 0g protein, 71.3g total fat, 1.4mg sodium, 0g fiber, <1mg calcium.

Onion-Infused Oil

What do you do with all the leftover white parts of scallions or leeks? Slice them into thin rounds, and freeze pieces in a zip-top bag to have on hand to make onion-infused oil.

½ cup chopped scallions, onions, or leeks, white
parts
½ cup extra virgin olive oil

- Follow directions as for garlic-infused oil. Store in a glass or ceramic container, tightly covered. Refrigerate garlic-infused oil immediately and discard after 4 days or freeze for long-term storage.

Yield: ⅓ cup

Substitutions: Any type of oil can be used in place of olive oil.

Nutrition (entire recipe): 630 calories, 0g carbohydrates, 0g protein, 71.3g total fat, 1.4mg sodium, 0g fiber, <1mg calcium.

Garlic- and Onion-Infused Oil

Lisa likes to make oil that is infused with both garlic and onion, since recipes often call for both flavors. The benefit of doing so is that you don't need to add each oil separately, which can add too much fat to a dish, and you can use up all of those scallion bulbs you've been accumulating.

8-10 peeled cloves garlic, coarsely chopped
½ cup chopped scallions, onions or leeks , white parts only
½ cup extra virgin olive oil

- Follow directions as for garlic-infused oil. Store in a glass or ceramic container, tightly covered. Refrigerate garlic-infused oil immediately and discard after 4 days or freeze for longer term storage.

Yield: ⅓ cup

Substitutions: Any other oil can be used in place of olive oil.

Nutrition (entire recipe): 630 calories, 0g carbohydrates, 0g protein, 71.3g total fat, 1.4mg sodium, 0g fiber, <1mg calcium.

Getting just the right heat—understanding chiles

It is a pleasant surprise for many people with IBS to discover they can enjoy spicy food again, once onions and garlic are out of the picture. Chili powder (note an "i" at the end of the word chili in this book) used to make chili con carne, is a blend of spices. It is made from one or more types of dried, ground chile peppers (note the "e" at the end of the word chile, used in this book to denote a single type of pepper) mixed with oregano, cumin, garlic and onion powder, and a few other spices. Cooking with individual chiles may be a new experience for you. You should know that chiles vary greatly in heat. You can customize chili powder to your heat preference by your selection of fresh or dried chiles:

No heat: paprika (unless labeled as hot)
Very mild: New Mexico, California
Mild: ancho, mulato, pasilla
Medium: cascabel
Medium hot: guajillo, chipotle, jalapeño
Hot: serrano
Very hot: chile de arbol, cayenne, pequin
Extremely hot: habanero, Scotch bonnet

Latin markets, independent natural food stores or well-stocked supermarkets often carry ground chile powder. Ordering chile powders online is an economical option, even with shipping, if you can't find single chile powders or chiles locally. Online sources of chile powder and whole, dried chile peppers include My Spice Sage, Whole Spice, Napa Valley, Penzey's, The Spice House, SpicesInc, and MexGrocer.com.

Chili Powder Mix

This low-FODMAP version omits the garlic and onion. The most commonly used chile in a chili powder mix is the relatively mild ancho chile. Chili Powder Mix can also be used to replace commercial taco seasoning mix, as most commercial blends contain garlic and onion powder.

6 tablespoons ancho chile powder
1-2 teaspoons chipotle chile powder
1 tablespoon smoked paprika
2 teaspoons ground coriander
3 tablespoons ground cumin
1 tablespoon dried oregano leaves
½ teaspoon ground black pepper
1 teaspoon asafetida (optional)

Tips: If you make Mexican food often, double or triple the recipe to keep on hand.

Variations: Other chile powders may be used in place of ancho if you prefer more heat.

- Stir spices together in a small bowl. Use immediately or store tightly covered for up to 6 months

Servings: 24, 1 teaspoon each. **Yield:** ½ cup

Nutrition (per serving): 11 calories, 1.8g carbohydrates, <1g protein, <1g total fat, 21.5mg sodium, 1g fiber, 17.2mg calcium.

Barbecue Spice Rub

If you like barbecue, you'll need this rub, because most commercial spice rubs contain garlic and onion powder. This low-FODMAP version adds barbecue taste to foods even when a grill isn't available.

2 tablespoons smoked paprika
2 tablespoons regular paprika
¼ cup packed light brown sugar
2 teaspoons salt
2 tablespoons ground ancho chile powder
1 teaspoon ground black pepper
2 tablespoons dry mustard powder
1 tablespoon ground cumin
1 tablespoon ground coriander seed
½ teaspoon asafetida powder (optional)
½ teaspoon ground chipotle chile powder
   (optional)

Substitutions: See discussion of chile powder substitutions (previous page) for various levels of heat.

Nutrition (per serving): 13 calories, 2.6g carbohydrates, <1g protein, <1g total fat, 146.6mg sodium, <1g fiber, 7.6mg calcium.

- Mix spices together. Store airtight, in a cool, dark place for up to 6 months.

Servings: 32, ½ tablespoons each. **Yield:** 1 cup

Barbecue Spice Paste

2 tablespoons Barbecue Spice Rub (above)
2 tablespoons garlic-infused oil
1 teaspoon liquid smoke (optional)

Nutrition (per serving): 74 calories, 2.7g carbohydrates, <1g protein, 7.1g total fat, 164mg sodium, <1g fiber, 7.8mg calcium.

- Combine spice rub, oil, and liquid smoke, if using. Brush all over food. Grill, broil, pan fry, or roast. This recipe makes enough for 1 pound of meat, chicken, or fish.

Servings: 4

Lisa's Ketchup

It's not as hard as it used to be to find ketchups sweetened with sugar instead of high-fructose corn syrup, but they still contain onions and garlic. Going without ketchup is difficult for some people, so this low-FODMAP ketchup might save the day. It comes very close to commercial brands in taste and texture. Do stay near the stove for frequent stirring to prevent the ketchup from burning. Karo Light Corn Syrup is not high-fructose corn syrup, and it is suitable for a low-FODMAP diet. See Substitutions if you'd prefer to make a brown sugar version.

1 tablespoon plus 1 teaspoon garlic-infused oil, divided
6 scallions, green part only, left whole
2 cups tomato puree with no added garlic or onion (do not use crushed tomatoes, tomato paste or tomato sauce)
6 tablespoons white vinegar
½ cup plus 1 teaspoon Karo Light Corn Syrup (not "Lite")
½ teaspoon dry mustard
1 bay leaf
⅛ teaspoon ground cloves
⅛ teaspoon ground ginger
¼ teaspoon allspice
¼ teaspoon coriander
¼ teaspoon paprika
¼ teaspoon ground black pepper
½ teaspoon salt
1 large pinch ground cinnamon
⅛ teaspoon asafetida

Tips: Freeze ketchup in an ice cube tray for ready access to small portions. When frozen, pop cubes into a zip-top bag. Use leftover tomato puree in soups, on pasta, or as a substitute for tomato paste in recipes. (Tomato puree is less concentrated than tomato paste, so use 2 times the amount of puree to paste.)

Substitution: 3 tablespoons packed light brown sugar and ⅓ cup of water can be used in place of Karo Light Corn Syrup. Brown sugar ketchup tastes great, but the color, texture and sweetness aren't quite the same as commercial ketchup.

Nutrition (per serving): 21 calories, 5.4g carbohydrates, <1g protein, <1g total fat, 118mg sodium, <1g fiber, 14.8mg calcium.

- Heat 1 tablespoon garlic-infused oil in a 2-quart saucepan. Sauté scallion greens until soft, 1-2 minutes, do not brown. Add tomato puree, vinegar, corn syrup, and spices and stir. Bring to a boil, reduce heat and simmer uncovered while stirring and scraping bottom and edges of pan with a rubber spatula every few minutes until ketchup is thick and reduced to 2 cups, 30-40 minutes. Pay attention to stirring near the end of cooking time to prevent burning. Remove scallion greens and bay leaf and discard. Stir in remaining 1 teaspoon garlic-infused oil.
- Store tightly covered in the refrigerator for up to four days or freeze for extended storage.

Servings: 16, 2 tablespoons each. **Yield:** 1 cup

Orange-Maple Dipping Sauce

Kids love "dipping." This tastes delicious on Oven-Fried Coconut Shrimp (page 88) or Chicken Nuggets (page 90).

¼ cup Lisa's Ketchup (above)
2 tablespoons orange juice
½ teaspoon orange zest
2 tablespoons 100% pure maple syrup
2 tablespoons mayonnaise
1 tablespoon white vinegar
⅛ teaspoon ground black pepper
⅛ teaspoon cayenne pepper (optional)

Nutrition (per serving): 49 calories, 8.9g carbohydrates, <1g protein, 1.7g total fat, 147mg sodium, <1g fiber, 10.6mg calcium.

- Whisk ingredients together in a small bowl until smooth. Serve immediately or keep up to four days in the refrigerator.

Servings: 6, 2 tablespoons each

Arugula Spinach Pesto

Pesto can be made with greens and is a great way to work extra vegetables into a dish. You may even get your kids to try "green pasta." Since raw garlic is not suitable for a low-FODMAP diet, garlic- and onion-infused oil combined with arugula's peppery bite provide the flavor. Makes a great topping for pizza, arepas, pasta, sandwiches, and burgers.

¾ cup walnut halves (3 ounces)
4 ½ cups baby arugula (5 ounces)
9 ½ cups baby spinach (6 ounces)
1 cup fresh basil leaves (1 ounce)
¼ cup finely chopped chives or scallion, green
 part only
1 cup grated Parmesan or Romano cheese (4
 ounces)
½ teaspoon salt
¼ teaspoon black pepper
1 teaspoon lemon zest
⅓ cup Garlic- and Onion-Infused Oil (page 124)

Tips: Use 1 cup pesto per pound of low-FODMAP pasta.

Substitutions: ¾ cup pecans or ½ cup pine nuts can be used in place of ¾ cup walnuts.

Nutrition (per serving): 93 calories, 1.6g carbohydrates, 3g protein, 8.7g total fat, 131mg sodium, <1g fiber, 75.8mg calcium.

- Pulse walnuts in a food processor until coarsely chopped. Add arugula, spinach, and basil leaves in batches and pulse until volume is reduced and leaves are coarsely chopped. Add chives, cheese, salt, pepper, zest, and pulse until a coarse puree forms. With machine running, drizzle in garlic- and onion-infused oil, until you have a puree with a little bit of texture. Refrigerate for up to 2 days, tightly wrapped, or freeze in airtight containers for 3-4 months.

Servings: 20, 2 tablespoons each. **Total yield:** 2 ⅔ cups.

Creamy Caesar Dressing

Don't fear the anchovy. It will add an authentic Caesar dressing taste without a fishy taste. Dressing tastes best when made an hour or more in advance.

½ cup mayonnaise
⅓ cup grated Parmesan cheese (1 ¼ ounce)
3 tablespoons fresh lemon juice
¼ cup lactose-free milk
1 anchovy filet
1 tablespoon garlic-infused oil
1 teaspoon Dijon mustard
½ teaspoon reduced-sodium soy sauce
¼ teaspoon granulated sugar
Several generous grinds black pepper

Tips: If not using a blender or food processor, use very finely grated Parmesan cheese for a smooth dressing.

Nutrition (per serving): 70 calories, 3.5g carbohydrates, 1.9g protein, 5.5g total fat, 110.3mg sodium, <1g fiber, 51mg calcium.

- Process all ingredients in a blender or food processor. Allow flavors to blend for at least 15 minutes. Serve the same day or refrigerate for up to 4 days.

Servings: 8, 2 tablespoons each

Gremolata

It doesn't get easier than this Italian condiment, which instantly pumps up the flavor of pasta, chicken, lamb, veal, fish, salads, or soup. Tossed onto foods just before serving, it adds a lot of flavor to cooked vegetables like zucchini, summer squash, and green beans. It is also great on baked potatoes, and in potato salad or pasta dishes.

Zest from 1 lemon
3 tablespoons finely chopped parsley leaves
2 tablespoons finely chopped chives or scallions,
    green part only
1 tablespoon garlic-infused oil
⅛ teaspoon salt
Few grinds of pepper

- Mix all ingredients in a small bowl. Allow flavors to blend for a few minutes before using. Serve the same day or refrigerate up to four days.

Servings: 3, 2 tablespoons each

"Lemon or orange zest can add a lot of flavor to foods. A workhorse kitchen gadget worth having for the low-FODMAP diet is a fine rasp grater (Microplane grater) which can zest a whole lemon or orange in under a minute and leave the white pith behind."

Tips: If you don't have a zester or a rasp, use a vegetable peeler to slice thin yellow strips of lemon peel using gentle pressure so that white pith underneath is not included. Mince very finely with a sharp knife.

Variations: Cilantro can be used in place of parsley. Add one or more of the following: 1 tablespoon minced, fresh rosemary or 2 tablespoons minced, fresh basil or oregano leaves; 2 minced anchovy filets (omit salt); 3 tablespoons minced pine nuts or almonds; 6 pitted, black or green olives, finely diced (omit salt).

Nutrition (per serving): 22 calories, <1g carbohydrates, <1g protein, 2.3g total fat, 49.7mg sodium, <1g fiber, 5.5mg calcium.

Ranch Dressing

Vegetables with Ranch Dressing make a great snack.

½ cup lactose-free cottage cheese
¼ cup lactose-free milk
3 tablespoons mayonnaise
¼ teaspoon dried oregano
1 teaspoon dry mustard powder (or 2 teaspoons
    prepared mustard)
2 teaspoons garlic-infused oil
Two large pinches granulated sugar
Several grinds black pepper
1 tablespoon plus 1 teaspoon white vinegar
½ teaspoon lemon zest (optional)
2 tablespoons minced chives or scallion, green
    parts only

- Puree cottage cheese in a blender until smooth, about 30 seconds. Add remaining ingredients (except chives) and blend. Pour into a bowl, stir in chives. Serve immediately or refrigerate up to 4 days.

Servings: 8, 2 tablespoons each

Nutrition (per serving): 45 calories, 1.9g carbohydrates, 2.1g protein, 3.2g total fat, 87.4mg sodium, <1g fiber, 19.6mg calcium.

Lemon Vinaigrette

Dressing can taste flat without garlic and onion, but this bold, tart dressing overcomes that. Herbs are left out of the basic recipe so you can customize the flavor; see Variations.

1 ½ teaspoons Dijon mustard
¼ cup fresh lemon juice (about 2 lemons)
¼ teaspoon salt
¼ cup plus 1 tablespoon extra-virgin olive oil
2 ½ teaspoons granulated sugar
½ teaspoon finely grated lemon zest (optional)
2 tablespoons water
Large pinch xanthan gum (optional)

- Shake ingredients together vigorously in a tightly covered glass jar. Use immediately or store in the refrigerator for up to one week; once fresh herbs, scallion greens or chives have been added, use or discard within four days.

Servings: 6, 2 tablespoons each

"Lemon Vinaigrette is a low-FODMAP kitchen staple. Not just for greens, it can also be used on grain salads like rice, quinoa, sorghum, and millet, or in potato salad. It also makes a great marinade for meat, chicken, fish, or seafood."

Tips: Xanthan gum thickens the dressing and prevents it from separating.

Variations: Italian: 1 teaspoon of dried basil, 1 teaspoon of dried oregano, 2 tablespoons chopped fresh parsley. Fall: ¾ teaspoon dried, crushed sage leaves and ¾ teaspoon dried thyme (great with roasted vegetables). Provence flavors: 1 teaspoon lightly chopped dried rosemary, ½ teaspoon dried thyme leaves, 1 teaspoon dried oregano. Spring: 1 teaspoon dried tarragon, 2 tablespoons fresh chopped parsley, 3 tablespoons finely minced chives or green part of scallion (great with chicken or seafood).

Nutrition (per serving): 110 calories, 2.7g carbohydrates, <1g protein, 11.3g total fat, 112.9mg sodium, <1g fiber, 2.2mg calcium.

Raspberry Vinaigrette

This colorful dressing will add pizzazz to your salads. It pairs especially well with salads that include goat cheese, toasted walnuts, pecans, or pepitas, and fresh fruit. Add cooked chicken for a dinner salad.

1 cup fresh or thawed frozen unsweetened
    raspberries
2 tablespoons sugar
2 teaspoons Dijon mustard
3 tablespoons red wine or balsamic vinegar
⅛ teaspoon salt
¼ cup canola oil
¼ teaspoon salt
4 tablespoons water

- Measure berries, sugar, mustard, vinegar and salt into a blender or food processor and blend until smooth, about 30-45 seconds. Slowly pour oil while blending. Thin dressing with 2-3 tablespoons of water if necessary, until dressing is pourable. Pour dressing through a sieve to get rid of seeds, pressing on puree with a rubber spatula. Taste and adjust flavors with sugar or vinegar, depending on the sweetness of the raspberries. Serve immediately or cover and refrigerate for up to four days.

Servings: 8, 2 tablespoons each

Substitutions: Other types of vinegar can also be used.

Nutrition (per serving): 87 calories, 6.1g carbohydrates, <1g protein, 7g total fat, 126.5mg sodium, 1g fiber, 6.9mg calcium.

10-Minute Salsa

All commercial salsas contain garlic and onions. This mildly spicy salsa will appeal to kids; it tastes like commercial brands from a jar. The salsa freezes well so make a double batch and freeze.

1 tablespoon plus 1 teaspoon garlic-infused oil, divided
Two large pinches asafetida (optional)
½ cup plus 2 tablespoons thinly sliced green part of scallion (about 4 scallions), divided
2 medium tomatoes (12 ounces), diced into ¼-inch pieces
1 tablespoon finely chopped canned chipotle chile in adobo sauce
¼ teaspoon salt
¼ teaspoon granulated sugar
1 tablespoon red wine vinegar
2 tablespoons minced cilantro leaves

- Heat 1 tablespoon of garlic-infused oil in a small skillet on medium heat. Stir in asafetida and ½ cup scallion greens and sauté 1 minute. Add tomatoes and juices, chipotle chile, and salt. Cook until tomatoes turn thick and soften, stirring periodically, about 4 minutes. Turn heat to medium-low and add sugar and 3 tablespoons water. Simmer while stirring until mixture is thick, about 3 minutes. Remove from heat; add vinegar and remaining 2 tablespoons scallion greens, remaining 1 teaspoon garlic-infused oil, and cilantro. Thin with water if necessary. Chill before serving. Store tightly covered in the refrigerator for up to four days.

Servings: 12, 2 tablespoons each

Tips: In a hurry? Chill the salsa quickly by placing it in the freezer for a few minutes before serving.

Substitutions: 1 (14.5 ounce) can diced tomatoes plus juices (no added onion or garlic) can be used in place of fresh tomatoes; omit 3 tablespoons of water. ½ teaspoon chipotle chile powder can be used in place of chile in adobo sauce.

Variations: For mild salsa, use ½ teaspoon ancho chile powder and ¼ teaspoon ground cumin in place of chile in adobo sauce. For a fresh, uncooked salsa, omit the water and combine the remaining ingredients in a bowl. Let flavors blend for 15 minutes. This will be much thinner than cooked salsa.

Nutrition (per serving): 26 calories, 3.7g carbohydrates, <1g protein, 1.3g total fat, 168mg sodium, 1g fiber, 27mg calcium.

Oven-Baked Breadcrumbs

This is a great way to use up dried out (but not stale tasting) bread, broken pieces, or the heels of bread. Freeze bread pieces in a zip-top bag until you have enough for a pan or two. Crumbs can also be made from cereals, pretzels, chips, or other crunchy snacks. To save time, make a large batch to use for multiple recipes instead of making them each time you need them.

6 slices of any low-FODMAP bread

- Preheat oven to 325° F.
- Stack several slices and cut into ½-inch pieces. Place cut bread in a single layer on a baking sheet. Bake until dry and light golden brown, turning once during baking, 15-20 minutes. Cool to room temperature. Pulse toasted bread in a food processor until crumbs are the desired texture. Larger, coarse pieces give more crunch. If breadcrumbs are still soft, return to oven and bake until dry and crisp, 5-10 minutes. Store crumbs in an airtight container in the pantry, refrigerator, or freezer.

Yield: 1 cup

Tips: If you don't have a food processor, place bread in a zip-top bag and close, leaving a small opening. Crush bread with a rolling pin or a saucepan bottom, until you have crumbs. If storing at room temperature, crumbs must be very dry or they will get moldy.

Nutrition (entire recipe): 436 calories, 78.6g carbohydrates, 13.6g protein, 7.1g total fat, 970.4mg sodium, 6.5g fiber, 106.9mg calcium.

Italian Crumbs

Make these easy breadcrumbs and you won't pay astronomical prices for hard-to-find specialty crumbs. They can be used for breading meat, topping casseroles, or sprinkling over pasta.

1 cup **Oven-Baked Breadcrumbs (previous page)**
1 ½ teaspoons dried basil
1 teaspoon dried oregano
½ teaspoon salt
½ cup grated Parmesan or Romano cheese (2 ounces)

* Mix together, cover tightly, and store in refrigerator or freezer

Servings: 12, 2 tablespoons each. **Yield:** 1 ½ cups

Variation: Just before using, add 2 tablespoons minced fresh parsley per ½ cup of breadcrumbs.

Nutrition (per serving): 54 calories, 6.8g carbohydrates, 2.8g protein, 1.7g total fat, 226.6mg sodium, <1g fiber, 68.4mg calcium.

Panko-Style Breadcrumbs

Foods with a panko crust are wonderfully light and crunchy; however, they are made from wheat flour. Crushed corn flake cereal makes a great substitute. Commercially prepared corn flake crumbs are crushed too finely to provide much crunch to your food. It takes just minutes to make your own and they keep for a long time.

6 ½ cups corn flakes

* Place corn flakes in a zip-top bag. Close the bag, leaving a tiny opening for air to escape. Crush the flakes with a rolling pin, the bottom of a heavy pan, or a large can, until you have coarse crumbs. Corn flake crumbs can be stored, airtight, at room temperature for several months.

Servings: 16, 2 tablespoons each. **Yield:** 2 cups

Substitutions: Corn Chex, or crispy rice cereal can be used instead of corn flakes.

Nutrition (entire recipe): 655 calories, 157.8g carbohydrates, 12.2g protein, .2g total fat, 1727.2mg sodium, 8.2g fiber, 5.5mg calcium.

Wild Blueberry Syrup

Small wild blueberries (often found frozen) have more intense berry flavor than the larger cultivated blueberries. Serve this syrup over pancakes. It also tastes great stirred into plain lactose-free yogurt.

1 teaspoon cornstarch
1 tablespoon cold water
1 ½ cups frozen wild blueberries
2 tablespoons granulated sugar
1 teaspoon lemon zest (optional)
¼ teaspoon vanilla

* Combine cornstarch and water in a small bowl to form a slurry. Set aside.
* Stir together blueberries, ¼ cup water, sugar, and zest in a small saucepan. Bring blueberries to a boil over medium heat and then turn heat down to a brisk simmer and cook, stirring occasionally, for 10 minutes, or until berries have released juices and thickened. Drizzle in the cornstarch slurry, while stirring, until syrup has thickened, 1-2 minutes. Remove from heat and stir in vanilla and optional lemon zest. Serve warm over pancakes.

Servings: 6

Tips: No need to thaw frozen blueberries for this recipe.

Substitutions: 6 ounces large, cultivated blueberries may be used in place of wild blueberries.

Nutrition (per serving): 36 calories, 8.2g carbohydrates, <1g protein, <1g total fat, 2.1mg sodium, <1g fiber, 4.5mg calcium.

Snacks and Smoothies

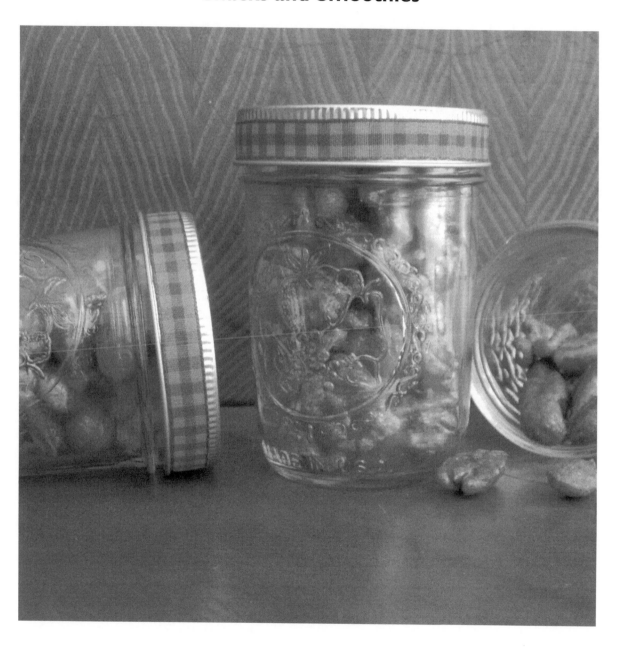

Candied Maple-Spiced Nuts

These glazed nuts can be sprinkled over a salad, or served as an appetizer or snack. You will need some parchment paper for this recipe.

3 cups raw nuts (combination of walnut halves, pecans halves, and whole almonds)
⅓ cup 100% pure maple syrup
½ teaspoon salt
1 teaspoon mild smoked paprika
½ teaspoon ground coriander
¼ teaspoon cayenne pepper

- Preheat oven to 350° F. Coat a baking sheet with baking spray or oil.
- Combine maple syrup, salt, smoked paprika, coriander, and cayenne pepper in a medium bowl. Add nuts and stir to coat.
- Scrape nuts and spices onto prepared pan in a single layer. Bake for 12-15 minutes, stirring halfway through baking. Nuts are ready when mixture is bubbling and syrup is almost dried up. Watch carefully during the last few minutes as the syrup can burn quickly.
- Remove nuts from the oven and immediately stir with a heatproof spatula to coat nuts with bubbling spice mixture. Transfer the nuts to a greased parchment paper. When cool, break up clumps of nuts, and store in an airtight container at room temperature for up to two weeks or longer in the refrigerator.

Servings: 24, 2 tablespoons each

Variations: ¾ teaspoon cinnamon or 1 ½ teaspoons curry powder can be used in place of paprika, coriander, and cayenne.

Nutrition (per serving): 108 calories, 5.1g carbohydrates, 2.3g protein, 9.6g total fat, 49.2mg sodium, 1g fiber, 17.8mg calcium.

Chocolate Banana Microwave Mug Cake

This cake is not for serving guests; it is a fun after-school snack or casual dessert that comes together fast when the craving strikes.

1 medium banana
1 large egg
2 tablespoons lactose-free milk
¼ teaspoon vanilla
⅓ cup Low-FODMAP All-Purpose Flour (page 57)
2 tablespoons unsweetened cocoa powder
1 tablespoon ground chia seeds or ½ tablespoon whole chia seeds
¼ cup granulated sugar
¼ teaspoon baking powder
2 tablespoons mini semi-sweet chocolate morsels
2 large pinches salt

- Mash banana in a small bowl. Stir in egg, milk, and vanilla. In one of the mugs, mix together the flour, cocoa powder, ground chia seed, sugar, baking powder, morsels, and salt. Pour flour mixture into the mashed bananas and stir until combined. Divide batter evenly between the two mugs. Microwave one mug at a time on high power for 1 minute. If batter looks wet, return to microwave for 15-second increments until cooked through. Total microwave time will be 1 -2 minutes. Enjoy eating from the mug or invert mug over a plate to remove cake. Cake is best eaten while warm.

Servings: 2

Tips: Microwave wattage, mug thickness, and depth of batter greatly affect cooking time. (Recipe was tested in a 1200 W microwave using 16-ounce mugs. Cooking time was 1 ½ minutes.)

Substitutions: If mugs aren't available, use 2 small microwaveable bowls.

Nutrition (per serving): 358 calories, 69.8g carbohydrates, 7.8g protein, 8.2g total fat, 400.3mg sodium, 6.1g fiber, 99.4mg calcium.

Peanut Butter Cup Nut Butter

Nut butter on bread, crackers, rice cakes, or bananas makes a quick, filling snack, but can be ho-hum. Flavored nut butters like this one kick it up a notch. Confectioners' sugar dissolves more readily in nut butter than does granulated sugar.

6 tablespoons confectioners' sugar
4 tablespoons plus 1 teaspoon unsweetened cocoa
    powder
½ cup creamy peanut butter
¼ teaspoon vanilla extract
4-6 tablespoons boiling water
Large pinch salt (if peanut butter is unsalted)

Substitutions: Granulated sugar can be used in place of confectioners' sugar, but reduce to 4 tablespoons. Add it to 4 tablespoons of the boiling water, stir to dissolve, and then proceed with recipe.

Nutrition (per serving): 167 calories, 14.3g carbohydrates, 6.2g protein, 11.4g total fat, 99.6mg sodium, 2.6g fiber, 14.3mg calcium.

- Stir the confectioners' sugar and cocoa powder together in a small bowl. Stir in peanut butter. It will be dry and pasty. Add vanilla and 4 tablespoons boiling water and stir until smooth, adding additional hot water if needed. Store the nut butter in an airtight container in refrigerator for several weeks.

Servings: 6, 2 tablespoons each

Maple Cinnamon Almond Butter

Maple extract is optional, but adds a more intense maple flavor.

½ cup almond butter
¼ heaping teaspoon cinnamon
3 tablespoons 100% pure maple syrup
¼ teaspoon vanilla extract
4 drops maple extract (optional)

Nutrition (per serving): 159 calories, 11.2g carbohydrates, 3.2g protein, 12.3g total fat, 94.7mg sodium, <1g fiber, 64.1mg calcium.

- Combine ingredients in a small bowl and stir until smooth.

Servings: 6, 2 tablespoons each

Banana Nut Butter "Sandwich"

Delicious, low-FODMAP variation on a classic snack.

½ banana
1 tablespoon Peanut Butter Cup Nut Butter or
    Maple Cinnamon Almond Butter (above)

Tips: Cut an unpeeled banana in half with a sharp knife and only peel the half you will be eating right away. Put the rest in the refrigerator to use next time. The skin will turn brown from the cold, but the banana inside will still be good for several days.

- Peel banana half and cut lengthwise. Spread one of the pieces with the flavored nut butter, then top with the other piece of banana to make a "sandwich."

Servings: 1

Nutrition (per serving): 74 calories, 8.3g carbohydrates, 2.3g protein, 4.2g total fat, 37.3mg sodium, 1.3g fiber, 4.9mg calcium.

Rice Cakes with Nut Butter and Fruit

Elevate the humble rice cake with a little nut butter love.

> **1 rice cake**
> **1 tablespoon Peanut Butter Cup Nut Butter or Maple Cinnamon Almond Butter (previous page)**
> **¼ cup blueberries**

- Spread a rice cake with 1 tablespoon of flavored nut butter. Spread blueberries across the peanut butter and press down slightly to get them to stick.

Servings: 1

Substitutions: Walnut, hazelnut, pecan, or sunflower seed butter can be used in place of flavored nut butter. Other low-FODMAP fruits can be used in place of blueberries, such as bananas or strawberries. Grated coconut can be used in place of fruit.

Nutrition (per serving): 150 calories, 15.7g carbohydrates, 5g protein, 1.7g total fat, 103.7mg sodium, 2.2g fiber, 10.1mg calcium.

Baked Corn Tortilla Chips

After putting out salsa for an after school snack one day, Lisa found that she was out of tortilla chips. After an "ah ha" moment, everyone was eating warm, crunchy, homemade chips made from baked, soft corn tortillas. Kids can cut the tortillas with a scissors into wedges, strips, circles, or random fun shapes. Keep pieces about 1-2 inches in diameter.

> **5 (6-inch) uncooked 100% corn tortillas**
> **¼ teaspoon salt**

- Preheat oven to 350° F.
- Lightly coat one side of each tortilla with baking spray or oil. Stack several tortillas and cut the stack with a knife into 8 wedges. Place individual pieces close together on a baking sheet, but not overlapping. Sprinkle with salt to taste. Bake until chips are crispy and golden on the bottom and lightly golden on top, 9-12 minutes. Chips will crisp up as they cool.

Servings: 4

Variations: For cinnamon sugar chips, combine ¼ cup sugar and 1 ½ teaspoons cinnamon and sprinkle as much as desired on tortilla chips in place of salt. For chili corn chips, sprinkle 1 ¾ teaspoons of Chili Powder Mix (page 125) on tortilla chips before baking. For curried tortilla chips, sprinkle chips with 1 teaspoon curry powder, ¼ teaspoon salt, and ¼ teaspoon sugar before baking.

Nutrition (per serving): 80 calories, 15.2g carbohydrates, 1.9g protein, 1.6g total fat, 148.9mg sodium, 1.7g fiber, 57mg calcium.

Why is corn syrup OK in low FODMAP recipes?
Before the 1970s, there was no such thing as high-fructose corn syrup. Old-fashioned corn syrup is not a source of excess fructose and provides just the right sweetness and stickiness for a successful granola bar. Read the label carefully when you purchase corn syrup—sometimes unwanted ingredients have been added. The recipes in this book call for Karo Light Corn Syrup, not "Karo Lite," which contains sucralose.

Granola Bar #25

Standard granola bars can be loaded with FODMAPs like inulin, chicory root fiber, wheat bran, honey, and dried fruits, so you may want to try making your own. Follow the recipe closely to get the right texture, as small changes make a big difference. Lisa has made this recipe 25 times to perfect it for you! Later, try some variations.

Oat Mixture:
2 ¼ cups uncooked old fashioned rolled oats
¼ cup brown rice flour
¼ cup uncooked millet seeds
¼ cup whole chia seeds
½ teaspoon cinnamon
⅓ cup salted, roasted peanuts, finely chopped
⅓ cup mini semi-sweet chocolate morsels
Sugar Syrup:
¼ cup packed light brown sugar
⅓ cup Karo Light Corn Syrup (not "Lite")
3 tablespoons canola oil
2 tablespoons water
1 teaspoon vanilla extract

- Preheat oven to 350° F. Generously coat a 9 x 9 x 2-inch pan with baking spray or oil. Coat a piece of foil slightly larger than the pan with baking spray or oil and set aside.
- Combine oats, flour, millet, chia, cinnamon, chopped nuts, and salt in a large mixing bowl.
- Measure brown sugar, corn syrup, canola oil, and 2 tablespoons water together into a small saucepan and stir just until sugar dissolves. Bring to a boil, turn heat down, and simmer for 1 minute. Remove from heat and stir in vanilla. Pour sugar syrup over oat mixture and stir until well mixed. Cool, stirring periodically, 4-5 minutes. Fold in chocolate morsels.
- Pour granola bar mixture evenly into prepared pan. Place foil, oiled side down, on top of the granola mixture. Press down on granola very firmly and evenly to pack tightly, paying attention to edges and corners. Set foil aside. Bake in the middle of the oven until the granola bars are lightly browned around the edges, 18-20 minutes.
- Remove pan from the oven and place the oiled side of foil on bars. Cover hand with an oven mitt and press down evenly and firmly on the bars to compact again. Remove foil and cool to room temperature. Invert pan over a cutting board, and rap on pan to release granola bar in one piece. Turn bar over, right side up. Cut bars into 18 pieces with a large knife using a gentle rocking motion. Store bars at room temperature with plastic wrap between layers or freeze for extended storage. Bars become softer and chewier over time.

Servings: 18

Tips: Coat cup with baking spray or oil before measuring Karo Syrup. Wrap bars individually in plastic wrap and refrigerate or freeze for up to several weeks.

Substitutions: Other sweeteners are not as successful in this recipe, but in a pinch you can use brown rice syrup or Lyle's Golden Syrup instead of Karo Light Corn Syrup. Maple syrup can be used in place of brown sugar (omit water). Walnuts, pecans, or almonds can be used in place of peanuts.

Variations: Add ⅓ cup shredded coconut.

Nutrition (per serving): 192 calories, 28.6g carbohydrates, 5.1g protein, 7.2g total fat, 22.8mg sodium, 4.1g fiber, 38.6mg calcium.

Peanut Butter Banana Smoothie

Peanut butter adds a shot of protein and healthy fat to this great-tasting smoothie.

2 tablespoons uncooked rolled oats
½ medium banana, preferably frozen, cut into
    several pieces
1 tablespoon peanut butter
2 teaspoons sugar
½ cup lactose-free milk
⅛ teaspoon vanilla

Nutrition (per serving): 346 calories, 53.7g carbohydrates, 12.6g protein, 11g total fat, 129.1mg sodium, 5.7g fiber, 167.8mg calcium.

• Grind oats to a powder in the blender. Add remaining ingredients and blend until smooth.

Servings: 1

Tofu "Almond Joy" Smoothie

Make this smoothie in advance and allow it to chill, since no frozen ingredients are added. Even Lisa's tofu-averse friends liked this smoothie.

2 tablespoons uncooked rolled oats
2 tablespoons toasted, finely shredded coconut
    flakes
1 tablespoon cocoa powder
4 ounces firm tofu, drained
1 ½ tablespoons granulated sugar
⅛ teaspoon almond extract
¼ teaspoon vanilla
1 cup canned light coconut milk
1 tablespoon coarsely chopped almonds
    (optional)

Tips:. Toast 1 cup coconut in a dry medium skillet on medium-low heat. Stir constantly until golden brown, 3-5 minutes. Or toast in a 350° F oven, 4-7 minutes, stirring 2-3 times. Or toast in microwave on high power for 30 second increments. Store toasted coconut in an airtight container for up to 2 months.

Nutrition (per serving): 521 calories, 40.6g carbohydrates, 18.6g protein, 35.9g total fat, 39mg sodium, 8.8g fiber, 338mg calcium.

• Grind oats to a powder in the blender. Add remaining ingredients except almonds. Blend until smooth, adding additional coconut milk if needed. Chill for 15-30 minutes, garnish with almonds, and serve.

Servings: 1

Strawberry Lemon Cheesecake Smoothie

The cottage cheese in this dessert-like smoothie will become completely smooth in the blender, so don't be afraid to try it.

1 tablespoon whole chia seeds
½ cup lactose-free cottage cheese
⅓ cup lactose-free milk
2-3 teaspoons granulated sugar to taste
¼ teaspoon vanilla
6 frozen strawberries (3 ounces)
1 ½ teaspoons fresh lemon juice
½ teaspoon lemon zest

• Grind chia seeds briefly in the blender. Add cottage cheese, milk, sugar, and vanilla to the blender and puree until smooth. Add strawberries, lemon juice, and zest and blend until smooth.

Servings: 1

Tips: Freeze your own fresh low-FODMAP fruit. Cut larger fruits into 1-inch pieces. Place fruit on a baking sheet with spaces in between pieces. When frozen, pop fruit into a zip-top bag.

Substitutions: ½ cup of frozen blueberries or raspberries can be used in place of strawberries. Almond or hemp milk can be used in place of lactose-free milk.

Nutrition (per serving): 264 calories, 31.9g carbohydrates, 19.9g protein, 6.9g total fat, 289.6mg sodium, 8.6g fiber, 270.9mg calcium.

Tips for sensational low-FODMAP smoothies

1. Use frozen fruit; it makes smoothies thick, creamy, and cold. Peel and quarter bananas. Store them in the freezer so you'll be ready to make a frosty smoothie at a moment's notice.

2. Freeze liquid ingredients like coconut milk in an ice cube tray in advance to cut back on chilling time. No need to thaw, just toss the frozen cubes right into the blender with the other ingredients

3. Add ingredients that have thickening power. Choose one or more of the following:

   • 2-3 tablespoons rolled oats; grind to a powder before adding other ingredients
   • 1 tablespoon chia seeds (whole or ground)
   • 2-4 ounces firm or extra firm tofu
   • 1-2 pinches xanthan gum (add to liquids, blend, then add remaining ingredients)

Refrigerate the smoothie for 5-10 minutes after making it to let the ingredients work their magic.

Lactose-Free Yogurt

Contrary to what many people believe, commercial yogurt is often high in lactose. It can range from 3-19g of lactose per cup, which can be more lactose than the 10-12g in a cup of milk! Long culture times result in yogurt that is low in lactose but with a tart taste, so manufacturers often culture milk for just a few hours. To make matters worse for those who can't tolerate lactose, milk solids, which are high in lactose, are often added to yogurt to thicken it, since the texture of yogurt in its natural state is quite thin. Greek-style yogurt is simply regular yogurt that has been drained of some of the lactose-containing whey, so it is often lower in lactose than regular yogurt.

The approximate lactose content of a *plain, unsweetened* commercial yogurt can be estimated by reading the Nutrition Facts Label on the container. Lactose is a sugar. The lactose present in yogurt will show up on the "sugars" line of the nutrition facts. For example, 4g of sugar means that the yogurt probably contains 4 grams of lactose per serving. If the yogurt is sweetened, it is not possible to determine whether the sugar comes from the lactose, added sweetener, or fruit. (This trick doesn't work for commercially produced lactose-free yogurt; when the milk is treated with lactase enzyme, lactose is converted to simpler sugars that still register as "sugars" on the nutrition facts.)

Since lactose-free yogurt can be hard to find, you may want to learn how to make your own. It is remarkably easy, takes only about 25 minutes to set up the cultures, and no yogurt maker is needed! It can be made from any percent fat, lactose-free cow's milk. Lisa prefers 1-2% or whole milk over non-fat milk for the richer, creamier taste without a lot more calories. Since homemade yogurt is thinner than supermarket yogurt and gets even thinner upon stirring, it is best not to stir it much after making it. Alternatively, it can be made thicker by adding a small amount of plain, unflavored gelatin before culturing, or by draining off the liquid to make thick Greek-style yogurt. Not only is homemade lactose-free yogurt economical, you can also control its thickness, sweetness, and flavor. Drained, unsweetened lactose-free yogurt can be used as a sour cream substitute, as a base for dips, or made into cheese, and the benefits of using yogurt in low-FODMAP baking cannot be overstated.

A heating pad is an easy, economical heat source for making yogurt, but make sure it does not have an automatic shut-off feature. Yogurt develops best between 110-115° F. Do not go above 115° F, or yogurt cultures may die or produce grainy yogurt. For those reasons, aim for 110° F. To test your heating pad, turn on the lowest setting for 10 minutes and place it on top of a folded towel. Cover pad with a thin towel. Fill a bowl or pot with 110-115° F. water, place on the heating pad and cover with plastic wrap or a lid. Cover everything with another towel. Check the water temperature with a quick-read or candy thermometer several times over a 1-2 hour period to see if it stays within the 110-115° F. range. If the water is too hot, leave an opening in the towel for heat to escape, or place another folded towel between the bowl and heating pad to lessen the direct heat; use both options if necessary. Re-check temperatures. Try the medium setting if the low setting is too cool.

Tools for making yogurt must be scrupulously clean. Use pots, bowls, or jars fresh out of the dishwasher. If you don't have a dishwasher, pour boiling water into pots and bowls and over utensils (do not submerge thermometer). Let sit for one minute, drain, and air dry. Wash hands and do not touch the inside of containers or the ends of utensils. Place plastic wrap or foil on counter to set down utensils. Sanitize the inside of the sink where you will later cool the milk in an ice and water bath.

Be sure that the plain commercial yogurt used as your starter lists "live active cultures" on the container, and is within the expiration date. Regular or Greek-style yogurt may be used, and it need not be lactose-free. Large name brands reliably have active cultures. Lisa has tried 3 major brands, with consistently good results.

8 cups (2 quarts) *lactose-free* milk (non-fat, 1%, 2%, or whole)
2 tablespoons plain unsweetened commercial yogurt
1 teaspoon granulated sugar
1 teaspoon unflavored gelatin powder, optional thickener (*do not use gelatin if you want to make Greek-style yogurt*)

Tips: Recipe can be halved or doubled. If you wish to ferment the cultured milk in smaller containers, pour it into stainless, ceramic, or glass bowls, or 1-2-quart glass jars. Cover containers with plastic wrap or lids and place on heating pad, then cover all with a towel or blanket. Leftover commercial yogurt

- Pre-warm heating pad to 110-115° F. Place pad on a folded towel and cover with a tea towel.
- Measure milk and sugar into a 3-quart pot on medium-high heat. If using gelatin, sprinkle it over the top of the milk and let it sit without stirring. Clip thermometer to pan so that the tip is not touching pan bottom or sides. After 5 minutes, stir milk every 2-3 minutes, just before reading temperature. Milk will stick slightly to the pan bottom, so when stirring be careful not to dislodge it or your yogurt will be lumpy. If milk is scorching, turn the heat down to medium. When milk reaches 185-190° F, about 10-15 minutes, turn off heat. Alternatively, heat milk in a large microwave safe bowl on high power in 2-3 minute increments, stirring and checking the temperature after each interval. Shorten heating time to 30-60 seconds as the milk nears temperature. If you do not have a thermometer, heat milk until it is steaming and foamy bubbles form around the edges of the pan. Do not boil.
- Cool milk to 110-115° F. To speed cooling, fill sink with cold water to the depth of milk in the pan and add several dozen ice cubes. Cover pot to prevent water splashing in, and place in the sink for 5-10 minutes. Remove cover and stir every few minutes to speed cooling.
- Add the commercial yogurt to milk. While milk is cooling, measure 2 tablespoons of commercial yogurt into a small bowl. When milk reaches 110-115° F, remove pan from sink and dry the outside. Add about 1 cup of warm milk to the yogurt while whisking. When smooth, stir diluted yogurt into the pot of warm milk.
- Keep cultured milk warm (110-115° F). Cover the pan and place on the heating pad. Important: leave cultured milk undisturbed for 6-12 hours while it ferments; jostling or moving containers can prevent setting. The longer the milk is fermented, the thicker and more tart the yogurt will be.
- After 6-12 hours gently tilt container to see if the milk has solidified. It will look like yogurt with its custard-like texture, and you may see whey, a yellowish liquid, on the surface of the yogurt. Taste, smell, and texture will tell you if you have yogurt. It should look like yogurt, smell like yogurt, and taste tart if it has set properly. If it smells or tastes bad or "off," smells like yeast or beer, has a stringy texture, or does not set up, throw it away and try again another time.
- To thicken yogurt by draining (optional, and only if gelatin was not used), line a large colander with a layer of overlapping paper towels, coffee filters, or clean unbleached muslin. Pour yogurt into lined colander and place it over a large bowl or pot with room below the colander for the whey to drain. Cover and refrigerate until the desired thickness is reached, 1-2 hours for thicker regular yogurt, 2-6 hours for Greek-style yogurt or sour cream-like product, or 12 hours to make a thick, cream cheese-like product suitable for dips. Drain 24 hours for yogurt cheese (a.k.a. labneh). Transfer yogurt from the colander into a clean covered container and refrigerate for up to 3 weeks.
- Refrigerate yogurt in the container for 3-4 hours before serving.

Servings: 8, 1 cup of undrained yogurt each. Yield decreases to 4-6 cups if drained.

can be covered tightly and refrigerated for 2-3 weeks to use as a starter to make more yogurt, if within the expiration date. Do not use homemade yogurt as a starter, as you may have a weaker culture and end up with a batch that does not turn into yogurt. Since the recipe started with lactose-free milk, drained whey from making Greek yogurt can be used as a liquid to replace milk or buttermilk in baking or added to soups.

Variations: Regular or thickened yogurt can be flavored or sweetened just before serving. Try ¼ teaspoon of vanilla, almond, maple, coconut, or coffee extract per cup of yogurt; stir in gently; try lemon or orange zest for citrus flavor; sweeten yogurt with fruit, sugar, maple syrup, stevia, sugar-sweetened jam, or Wild Blueberry Syrup (page 131).

Nutrition for undrained yogurt made with low-fat milk (per serving): 110 calories, 2.5g total fat, 125mg sodium, 13g carbohydrates, 0g fiber, 8g protein, 300mg calcium.

Soups

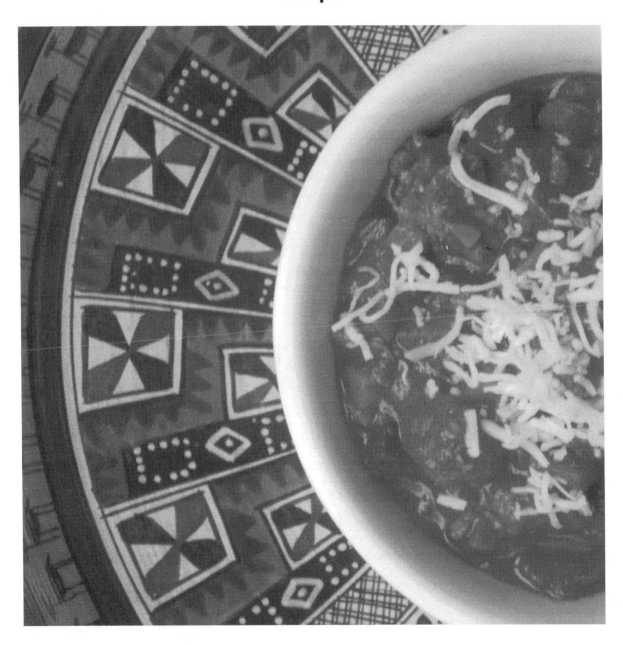

Chili Soup

This dish is delicious, either with or without the addition of Cornmeal Dumplings (below).

> 1 pound extra-lean ground beef or turkey
> 1 tablespoon garlic-infused oil
> 5 scallions, green part only, sliced thinly
> 1 large red bell pepper, seeded and diced into ¼-inch pieces
> 1 tablespoon cumin
> 1 tablespoon ancho chile powder
> ½ teaspoon asafetida (optional)
> 1 teaspoon salt
> ¼ teaspoon freshly ground black pepper
> 1 teaspoon smoked paprika
> 2 cups canned tomato puree (no added onions or garlic)
> 4 cups Lisa's Chicken Stock (page 146) or water
> 2 cups water
> 4 ounces peeled rutabaga, diced into ¼-inch pieces
> 2 cups peeled, ½-inch diced butternut squash
> 1 yellow summer squash (½ pound), diced into ¼-inch pieces
> 1 zucchini (½ pound), diced into ¼-inch pieces
> 1 cup grated sharp cheddar cheese (4 ounces)
> Sour cream (optional)

Tips: If you are unable to purchase at least 90% lean ground beef or turkey, drain the browned meat before proceeding with the recipe.

Nutrition calculated using water, without dumplings (per serving): 257 calories, 11.8g carbohydrates, 16.3g protein, 16.7g total fat, 526.4mg sodium, 3.4g fiber, 174.3mg calcium.

- Sauté ground beef in a large Dutch oven or stock pot. Chop it into small pieces until meat is no longer pink and is well browned. Add garlic-infused oil, scallion greens, and bell pepper and sauté until softened, about 2-3 minutes. Stir in cumin, ancho chile powder, asafetida, salt, pepper, and smoked paprika and sauté one minute. Add tomato puree, chicken stock, 2 cups water, rutabaga, and butternut squash. Simmer covered for 15 minutes. Stir in yellow squash and zucchini, cover, and cook until vegetables are soft but not mushy, about 10 minutes.
- Divide soup into bowls, topping each with 3 tablespoons grated cheddar cheese. Top each with 2-3 cornmeal dumplings (optional) and a dollop of sour cream or Greek yogurt.

Servings: 8

Cornmeal Dumplings

Whip up these easy dumplings while your Chili Soup simmers to make it a complete meal.

> ½ cup lactose-free milk
> ½ teaspoon vinegar
> 1 cup yellow cornmeal
> 1 ¼ cup Low-FODMAP All-Purpose Flour (page 57)
> 1 ½ teaspoons baking soda
> ¼ teaspoon salt
> 2 eggs
> 2 tablespoons canola or olive oil

Nutrition (per serving): 187 calories, 30g carbohydrates, 4.6g protein, 5.7g total fat, 351.2mg sodium, 2.1g fiber, 29.5mg calcium.

- Bring a large covered pot of water plus 1 tablespoon salt to a boil. Add ½ teaspoon vinegar to a liquid measuring cup. Fill with milk up to the ½-cup mark and set aside.

- Combine cornmeal, flour mix, baking soda and salt in a medium bowl.
- Beat eggs in a small bowl. Add eggs and milk to dry ingredients and stir to combine. Use a teaspoon to scoop up a golf-ball-sized portion of batter. Use a second teaspoon to scrape the dumpling into the boiling water. Repeat until all dumplings are formed. Turn heat down to maintain a low boil, loosening any dumplings that stick to the bottom. Cook for about 10 minutes. To test for doneness, cut a dumpling through the center. The middle should be bread-like and not doughy. Spoon dumplings into a colander to drain.

Servings: 8, 3 dumplings each

Creamy Fall Root Vegetable Soup

This smooth soup is surprisingly kid-friendly and it is easy to make.

1 tablespoon butter or garlic-infused oil
1 ½ cup rutabaga (½ pound) peeled and cut into
  ½-inch pieces
3 large parsnips (¾ pound), peeled and cut into
  ½-inch pieces
3 large carrots (¾ pound), peeled and cut into ½-
  inch pieces
1 large russet potato (¾ pound), peeled, cut into
  1-inch pieces
1 large sweet potato (¾ pound), peeled, cut into 1-
  inch pieces
⅓ cup thinly sliced leek leaves, green part only
4 cups Lisa's Chicken Stock (page 146) or water
2 cups water
1 teaspoon dried thyme
½ teaspoon dried sage leaves, crumbled
1 dried bay leaf
½ teaspoon asafetida (optional)
1 teaspoon salt
Several generous grinds of pepper
3 cups lactose-free milk
½ cup heavy or whipping cream

- Melt butter in a Dutch oven or a large stockpot on medium-high heat. Add rutabaga, parsnips, carrots, and potatoes in a single layer and cook undisturbed until browned, 3-4 minutes. It may be necessary to do this in two batches. Stir and turn vegetables over to allow vegetables to brown on another side for a few minutes. If cooking in two batches, remove browned vegetables from pot, add remaining vegetables and brown. Return all vegetables to pot, along with leek leaves. Stir periodically for 2-3 minutes. Add 4 cups chicken stock or water, 2 cups water, thyme, sage, bay leaf, asafetida, salt, and pepper. Cover pot, bring to a boil, and reduce heat to a simmer. Cook until vegetables are soft and easily pierced with a knife, 35-40 minutes.
- Turn off heat and remove bay leaf.
- Pour in milk and puree soup with an immersion blender, or in batches in a blender or food processor. Return soup to the pot and add cream. Soup should be thick, smooth, and creamy. Stir and adjust taste with salt and pepper. Add additional milk or water if necessary.

Servings: 8

Tips: Browning foods is a useful flavor-building technique that allows the natural sugars in foods to caramelize. Use this technique often in cooking when pan-frying, broiling, or roasting, where the high heat will do the work for you.

Variations: Omit thyme and sage and add 1 tablespoon curry powder. Instead of pan browning vegetables, roast them in a 425° F oven until lightly browned, about 25 minutes, turning once.

Nutrition calculated using all water (per serving): 218 calories, 31.5g carbohydrates, 6g protein, 8.2g total fat, 461.4mg sodium, 4.9g fiber, 185.9mg calcium.

Lisa's Chicken Stock

One of our recipe testers calls this stock "Lisa's Delicious Healing Elixir" because it is so tasty, rich, hydrating and healthy! Most commercial stocks contain onions. Lisa found that leek greens, which are suitable for a low-FODMAP diet, add oniony goodness to homemade stock. Prepping the stock takes only a few minutes, and it can be left simmering for hours without any hands-on effort. It is not necessary to peel vegetables if they are well scrubbed. Inexpensive chicken wings or legs make the most flavorful stock.

> 4 pounds chicken wings (or a combo of wings, legs, and backs)
> 2 carrots cut into large pieces
> 2 parsnips cut into large pieces
> ½ cup diced celery root/celeriac
> 2 leeks, green portion only
> 12 whole black peppercorns
> 2 teaspoons salt
> 2 dried bay leaves
> 10 sprigs fresh parsley
> 1 teaspoon dried thyme (or 8-10 fresh sprigs)
> 1 teaspoon dried sage leaves (not powder)
> 2 quarts water (approximately)

- Combine all dry ingredients in a Dutch oven or large stockpot. Add cold water just to cover ingredients. Cover pot, turn heat to medium-high and bring to a boil. Reduce heat to maintain a low simmer and cook for 3-6 hours. If stock cannot maintain a low bubble covered, tilt the lid slightly askew. Strain broth through a colander into a large container and chill overnight. Remove solidified fat from the surface with a spoon. Stock will keep refrigerated for 3-4 days or several months in the freezer.

Yield: 14 cups

Tips: Freeze the white parts of the scallion for future use in making onion-infused oil. Freeze stock in 1 and 2 cup portions so you can use it in small amounts. Freeze in even smaller amounts in an ice cube tray to add a few tablespoons of stock to a recipe. Once frozen, pop out of tray and store in a zip-top bag. If you have extra time, browning the vegetables before making the stock adds big flavor. Dice vegetables until they are the size of corn kernels. Brown in the stock pot on medium-high heat with 2 tablespoons of oil until medium golden brown, 8-10 minutes, stirring every few minutes. Add remaining ingredients and proceed with recipe.

Substitutions: Green part of scallion from 1 ½ bunches can be used in place of greens from 2 leeks.

Nutrition (entire recipe): 1210 calories, 118.6g carbohydrates, 84.7g protein, 40.3g total fat, 5423.8mg sodium, 0g fiber, 101mg calcium.

Chili Con Quinoa

Chili con carne with beans was a favorite of Lisa's family. Beans are high in FODMAPs, but chili without beans had the wrong texture. Adding quinoa and squash fixes this problem. Most commercial chili powder contains garlic and onion powder, so be sure to make your own using the recipe in this book.

> 1 tablespoon garlic-infused oil
> 2 pounds extra-lean ground turkey or beef
> ¼ cup Chili Powder Mix (page 125)
> 2 (14.5 ounce) cans petite diced tomatoes
> 1 ¼ teaspoons salt
> ½ teaspoon ground black pepper
> 6 scallions, green part only, sliced
> 1 cup quinoa, rinsed
> 2 cups peeled butternut or kabocha squash, cut into ½-inch chunks
> 3 ½ cups water

- Heat oil on medium-high heat in a large Dutch oven or stockpot. Add ground meat and stir, breaking up meat. When meat is no longer pink, add chili powder and sauté one minute. Add tomatoes, salt, pepper,

Tips: Butternut or kabocha squash can be peeled with a vegetable peeler. If you are unable to purchase at least 90% lean ground beef or turkey, drain the browned meat before proceeding with the recipe.

Substitutions: Millet can be used in place of quinoa; increase cooking time by 5-10 minutes.

scallion greens, quinoa, squash, and water. Cover pot and turn down to a simmer for 30 minutes. If mixture is too thick, add extra water.

Servings: 12

Nutrition (per serving): 284 calories, 36.3g carbohydrates, 19.7g protein, 9.8g total fat, 377.1mg sodium, 11.7g fiber, 189.5mg calcium.

Minestrone Soup with Garlic Toasts

Minestrone soup is a great way to get those who are vegetable-wary to eat their vegetables. This soup traditionally has cannellini or kidney beans, which are higher in FODMAPs; use canned, well drained, rinsed lentils instead.

Soup:
2 tablespoons garlic-infused oil
1 carrot, peeled and finely diced
1 medium parsnip, peeled and finely diced
½ cup thinly sliced leek leaves or chopped
    scallions, green part only
4 cups Lisa's Chicken Stock (previous page) or
    water
5 cups water
1 (14 ounce) can diced tomatoes
1 cup canned tomato puree
1 (14-ounce) can lentils, drained and rinsed
1 large russet potato (¾ pound), peeled and diced
    into ½-inch pieces
2 teaspoons dried basil
1 ½ teaspoons dried oregano
1 dried bay leaf
1 teaspoon salt
½ teaspoon black pepper
1 large zucchini (¾ pound), cut into ¼-inch
    pieces
½ pound green beans, cut into 1-inch pieces
1 ½ cups small low-FODMAP pasta (rice, corn, or
    quinoa)
Garlic Toasts:
2 slices low-FODMAP bread
2 tablespoons garlic-infused oil
Garnish:
½ cup grated Parmesan cheese (2 ounces)

Substitutions: 1 ½ cups cooked millet or quinoa or a 15-ounce can of rinsed, drained chick peas can be used in place of canned lentils.

Variations: Add 3 cups of baby spinach or sliced chard leaves in the last 5 minutes of cooking.

Nutrition calculated using water (per serving): 373 calories, 59.3g carbohydrates, 15.8g protein, 8.5g total fat, 449mg sodium, 17.8g fiber, 137mg calcium.

- Heat 2 tablespoons olive oil in a large Dutch oven on medium-low heat. Add carrot, parsnip, and leek tops. Sauté, stirring occasionally until vegetables soften and turn light golden brown, 8-10 minutes. Add chicken stock, water, diced tomatoes with juices, tomato puree, lentils, potato, basil, oregano, bay leaf, salt, and pepper. Turn heat to medium-high, bring to a boil, and lower heat to a simmer for 15 minutes. Stir in zucchini, green beans and pasta, cover and simmer until pasta is done, 15-20 minutes.
- While soup is simmering, brush both sides of bread with 2 tablespoons garlic-infused oil. Broil bread on both sides until golden brown. Slice bread into quarters. To serve, sprinkle each bowl of soup with 2 tablespoons grated Parmesan cheese, then top with 2 pieces of garlic toast. Pass additional Parmesan cheese with soup.

Servings: 10

APPENDIX

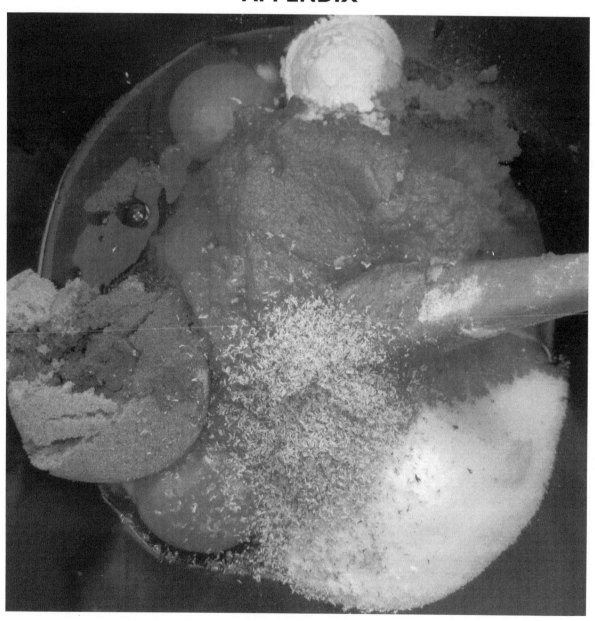

Weights, Volumes, and Measures

Weights and measures are very important to the success of your recipes. Unless you are a brilliant chef with terrific visual memory, you will not be able to estimate a cup of millet flour or a tablespoon of milk with any accuracy. Trust us. If you don't already own them, get yourself a nice set of measuring spoons, nesting measuring cups (for solids), and liquid measuring cups in 8-, 16-, and 24-fluid ounce sizes. Particularly in baking, the proportion of various ingredients must be carefully balanced to get the desired outcome. Make it a rule to follow recipes as closely as possible the first time you make them. If you must make substitutions, follow the guidance in the recipes and try to match the weights, volumes, and measures as closely as possible.

All of the "cups" used in this book refer to United States cups. Metric cups, used in many parts of the world, are slightly larger than United States cups. Cups, tablespoons, and teaspoons are meant to be loosely filled with the food to be measured, and a straight-edge should be scraped across for a level top. If you pack the food in (brown sugar is the only exception), or allow it to heap up over the top of the cup, your measurement will not be accurate, and your recipes will suffer. There are several excellent videos on YouTube about how to weigh and measure ingredients; consider watching them if you've never given this much thought. Here are some common equivalents:

1 ounce (oz) = 28.4 grams (g)
1 pound (lb) = 454 grams (g)
1 fluid ounce (fl oz) = 2 tablespoons (Tb) of liquid = 30 milliliters (ml)
1 quart (qt) = 32 fluid ounces (fl oz) = 960 milliliters (ml)
1 gallon (gal) = 64 fluid ounces (fl oz) = 1.9 liters (L)
1 cup (c): the *weight* of one cup of food depends on what the food is. One cup of butter weighs much more than one cup of crispy rice cereal, for example.
1 cup (c) = 240 ml. The *volume* of a cup of food does not vary. 1 United States cup is always 240 ml, which is a little smaller than a metric cup (250 ml).
1 tablespoon (T or Tb) = 3 teaspoons (t) = 15 milliliters (ml) ; tablespoons and teaspoons can be used to measure either solids or liquids.
1 teaspoon (t) = 5 milliliters (ml)
½ teaspoon (t) = 2.5 milliliters (ml)
¼ teaspoon (t) = 1.25 milliliters (ml)

Food Language for Global Cooks

People around the world suffer from IBS, and cooks around the world need to prepare food for them. This cookbook was written in the United States, but the terms for some foods and food preparation techniques are different elsewhere. The following is a review of terms used in this book and their foreign equivalents.

Appetizer is also known as starter
Arugula is also known as rocket
Baking soda is also known as bicarbonate of soda
Bell pepper is also known as a sweet pepper or capsicum
Butternut squash is also known as butternut pumpkin
Canned is also known as tinned
Cantaloupe is also known as a rockmelon
Cilantro is also known as coriander leaf
Confectioner's sugar is also known as icing sugar or powdered sugar
Cookies are also known as biscuits
Corn syrup is also known as glucose syrup
Cornmeal is also known as maize flour
Cornstarch is also known as cornflour
Dessert is also known as pudding or afters

Eggplant is also known as aubergine

Endive is also known as chicory or witloof

Chick peas are also known as garbanzo beans

Granulated sugar is also known as table sugar, white sugar, or sucrose

Green onions are also known as spring onions or scallions

Grilling is also known as barbecuing

Ground meats are also known as minced meats

Ketchup is also known as tomato sauce

Muffin is also known as quick bread

Peanuts are also known as ground nuts

Raisins are also known as sultanas

Raw shrimp are also known as green shrimp

Rice flour is also known as ground rice

Rutabaga is also known as swede or turnip

Sausages are also known as bangers

Shredded coconut is also known as desiccated coconut

Shrimp are also known as prawns

Skillet is also known as frying pan

Slice of bacon is also known as rasher of bacon

Sole is also known as bream

Spatula is also known as a fish slice

Stew beef is also known as gravy beef

Stove is also known as range

Stove burner is also known as hob

Summer squash is also known as yellow or crookneck squash

Swiss chard is also known as silverbeet

Tomato sauce is also known as pasta sauce

Tuna is also known as tunny

Zucchini is also known as courgette (immature) or marrow (mature)

ACKNOWLEDGMENTS

From Lisa: A special thank-you to my children, Isabel and Zachary, who patiently waited for many late meals, for their willingness to try new foods, for rating the meals with a kid-friendly "thumbs up" or "thumbs down," and for enduring the 25 trials of granola bars in lunch boxes with smiles and little eye-rolling. To my husband, Paul, who graciously eats everything I make, and who offered the adult approval or disapproval for recipes: Paul, thank you for running to the supermarket at all hours when I ran out of ingredients, and most importantly for washing the dishes when the sink overflowed, and I was too busy cooking or writing to help, and for cheering from the sidelines.

To all of my friends, I appreciate you for your support and encouragement to publish this cookbook, and for allowing me to turn every social event into a chance to taste, rate and taste again many of the recipes.

Thank-you to Karen Warman, RDN, for introducing me to the low-FODMAP diet and joining the project early on, even before we had a firm idea for how we would publish.

To Patsy Catsos, RDN, who jumped in as a collaborator and created order out of disorder, allowing this cookbook to become a reality. Thank you for having faith in my recipes early on, and for the beautiful photography in the book.

A special thank-you goes to my mother, Laura Rothstein, an adventurous cook who taught me how to cook at the tender age of five. She taught me traditional recipes and ethnic cooking, in addition to vegetarian cooking that she learned from the first vegetarian cookbooks in the early 70s, before it was even a fad. And to my father, Charles Rothstein, Ph.D., who taught me perseverance, instilled the idea that I would excel at what I loved to do, and encouraged me to find and pursue that which made me happy.

From Patsy: My family and friends got a little bit of a break from recipe testing during this project, since all of the wonderful recipes in this book were developed by Lisa. Few of us are as creative and technically accomplished in the kitchen as Lisa. Her persistence with problem solving is unbelievable and is a tribute to her background as a scientist. She thinks nothing of adjusting and retesting recipes repeatedly until they reach her high standard for just the right flavor, form, texture, color and aroma. Thank you, Lisa, for sharing the fruits of your labor with us.

Karen is a dedicated advocate for her pediatric patients, and she helped set the direction for this cookbook. She recognized the need for recipes and materials that could be used by families trying to cope with a diagnosis of IBS along with all the other family pressures of meal planning, school, work, tight budgets, and social lives. Thank you, Karen, for finding a way to make your vision a reality and for your contributions to this book.

Julie Salerno, thank you for your help with calculating the nutrient composition of the recipes. Lorie Catsos, Christy Catsos and Jennifer Caven provided editorial assistance, for which I am grateful. The last hands to touch the manuscript are mine, as editor, so I am responsible for any mistakes that crept in after they ably did their work. Collaborating on a book project and serving as editor for other writers was a new experience for me. I'd like to thank my dear husband, Paul, for his loving support, encouragement and assistance in navigating this new process.

I learn new things about digestive health every day from my patients, my referring physicians, my readers and from the dietitians with whom I work and train. I can scarcely express my gratitude to those of you who have taken the time to exchange ideas with me, review my books on Amazon.com, share my work with others, and help get the word about FODMAPs to IBS sufferers everywhere. I am particularly grateful to pre-publication reviewers of this book, including Ann Miranda, Colleen Francioli, Kasey Kaufman, Shalimar Poulin, Stephanie Carlson, and Ilene Cohen. I sincerely thank fellow members of the Academy of Nutrition and Dietetics who have shared their publishing wisdom and experience with me. Finally, closer to home, I am grateful for the support, encouragement and friendship of present and past members of the Maine Academy of Nutrition and Dietetics and to Susan Quimby and the rest of the staff at Nutrition Works LLC in Portland, Maine. Thank you for believing in me.

From Karen: I would like to acknowledge and thank the many families who permitted me to assist in their nutrition care. I have been privileged that families and like-minded professionals have supported my enthusiasm for raising awareness about FODMAPs. I am thankful to have two co-authors, Lisa and Patsy, whose expertise and passion for this subject has made the creation of a healthy family-oriented book a reality rather than a dream. Finally, I thank my own family, Matt, Marlee, and Ethan, who encourage and support my passion for providing nutrition care to families.

ABOUT THE AUTHORS

Lisa Rothstein holds a B.A. in Biology and was a cancer research scientist at Harvard Medical School and Dana Farber Cancer Institute for 17 years. During a second career she developed educational programs and resources for an infertility nonprofit organization.

Lisa has had a lifelong passion for cooking and healthy eating, and was a "foodie" well before the word existed. Ever curious about different ingredients and flavors, she stared down her first blocks of tofu and tempeh back in 1975 and found ways to make them tasty at the cusp of the health food craze.

After she was diagnosed with IBS as a teen, Lisa suspected that her symptoms were related to diet. Dietary recommendations from the medical community, however, only made her IBS worse, and she looked to other dietary changes for symptom improvement. Several years of eating a vegetarian diet did not offer relief, though it did further her cooking skills. In the 1980s she discovered that eating wheat- and lactose-free foods lessened her IBS symptoms. However, the very few wheat-free recipes and commercial foods that existed at that time were high in fat and nutritionally-deficient carbohydrates. After lots of experimentation, she developed healthier recipes using alternative whole grains and flours and became known in her community as an expert in these diets. Living and working in a multicultural environment, Lisa expanded her cooking repertoire to include Middle Eastern, Hispanic, and Asian cuisines, gaining knowledge of the unique foods and spices of these cultures.

When her IBS symptoms spiraled out of control, Lisa looked to the latest research for the Holy Grail of IBS management. In 2011, on a recommendation from dietitian Karen Warman, she explored the low-FODMAP diet and found that it dramatically reduced her symptoms. However, she realized that this diet required a lot of culinary creativity and careful meal planning. Combining the wide range of cooking and recipe development skills gained over the years, she is now devoting her time to creating healthy and tasty low-FODMAP recipes that appeal to both adults and children with IBS.

Lisa is a dilemma-free omnivore and resides in the greater Boston area with her husband, two children, and a very well-used kitchen.

Patsy Danehy Catsos, MS, RDN, LD, is a nutritionist on a mission to reduce pain and improve quality of life for people with digestive health issues, especially irritable bowel syndrome (IBS) and small intestinal bacterial overgrowth (SIBO). Patsy doesn't believe in one-size-fits-all diets; she aims to help you discover the diet that works for you.

Her trailblazing book, *IBS—Free at Last!* (Pond Cove Press, 2009), introduced U.S. health care providers and consumers to an exciting and effective dietary program for finding and eliminating food triggers for irritable bowel syndrome. Patsy is the editor of the blog IBSfree.net. She has been consulted for expert comments in numerous web and print publications, including *WebMD, Environmental Nutrition, Today's Dietitian, SpryLiving.com, Bloomberg.com, Blisstree.com, EmpowHer.com, CatchingHealth.com, Clinical Nutrition Insight* and *Consumer Reports Shop Smart Magazine*. Patsy provides continuing professional education internationally to other dietitians on the delivery of the FODMAP elimination diet.

Ms. Catsos earned a B.S. in Nutritional Science at Cornell University and an M.S. in Nutrition at Boston University. She completed her internship at Boston's Beth Israel Hospital. Ms. Catsos maintains a private practice in Portland, Maine. She is a professional member of the Crohn's and Colitis Foundation of American and the Academy of Nutrition and Dietetics, and she is a past president of the Maine Academy of Nutrition and Dietetics.

Patsy looks forward to corresponding with readers through her blog, www.ibsfree.net/news. Subscribe to the blog to get new posts delivered to your inbox. Follow @CatsosIBSFreeRD on Twitter, pcatsos on Pinterest and "like" IBSFree on Facebook to be notified about new blog posts, FODMAP-friendly foods, and other items of interest.

Karen Warman, MS, RDN, LDN, holds a Master's degree in Nutrition from Texas Woman's University and has been a registered dietitian for 34 years. She has worked as a clinical nutrition consultant helping clients with celiac disease, inflammatory bowel disease and irritable bowel disease at Johns Hopkins University, Children's National Medical Center, and Rainbow Babies and Children's Hospital. She is currently at Boston Children's Hospital in the Division of Gastroenterology and Nutrition.

Her career has focused on translating diet and nutrition information into meal plans and strategies that assist clients in improving their health. Many of her clients report that they are unskilled in the kitchen, but find reliance on prepackaged foods limits variety in their diet. Teaming up with Lisa and Patsy has resulted in a unique opportunity to combine nutrition knowledge with culinary skills and provide a complete package to those suffering with IBS.

INDEX

16387597R00096

Printed in Great Britain
by Amazon